regional
Human Anatomy
WORKBOOK

Steven E. Bassett
Southeast Community College
SECOND EDITION

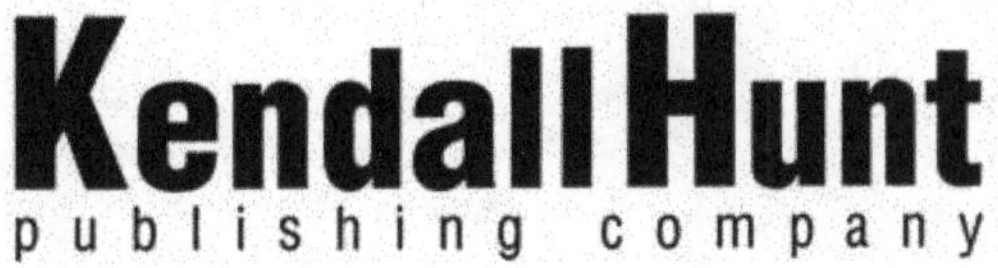

Kendall Hunt
publishing company

Cover image © Shutterstock, Inc.

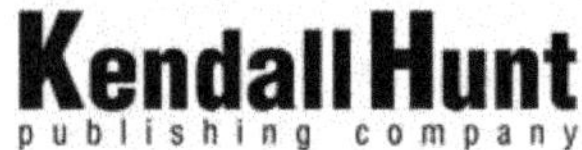

www.kendallhunt.com
Send all inquiries to:
4050 Westmark Drive
Dubuque, IA 52004-1840

Copyright © 2012, 2013 by Steven E. Bassett

Revised Printing 2014

ISBN 978-1-4652-5319-4

Printed in the United States of America

TABLE OF CONTENTS

I would like to thank my family, especially my wife, for being so understanding and supportive as I sit with the computer on my lap for several hours every night developing this workbook. She is very understanding in the sense that she knows while I am typing, I am only pretending to watch the television program she has on, which was usually some sort of sobbing love story.

I would also like to thank Hank Hinrichs and Elijah Knight for their expert input regarding this manual in reference to maintaining accuracy as much as possible.

I would also like to thank the wonderful people at the Kendall Hunt Publishing department. I thank them for the beautiful artwork on the cover page and also for putting up with all my emails regarding, "please make this change and that change before it goes to print."

I want to point out that the terms used in this manual are in accordance with the national anatomical society. The information in this manual strives to use anatomical terms and not layman's terms.

It is my intention that this manual will take rather difficult information and organize it in an understandable and usable format for the ease of the study and appreciation for the fantastic field of HUMAN ANATOMY.

Chapter 1:   Introductory Terminology

BODY TERMINOLOGY

In order to understand the anatomical terms associated with the superficial landmarks of the body, one must understand the directional terminology associated with human anatomy. The following table lists the directional terms that will be used in this course. In order to use the directional terms properly, one must first understand the anatomical position of the body. The **anatomical position** is where the body is in a standing position, feet together with the arms to the sides and the palms facing anterior (front).

Directional Terms

	Directional Term	Description	Example
1	**Superior**	Moving toward the head	The nose is superior to the lips.
2	**Inferior**	Moving toward the feet area	The chin is inferior to the lips.
3	**Lateral**	Moving away from the midline of the body	The thumbs are lateral to the index finger.
4	**Medial**	Moving toward the midline of the body	The big toe is the most medial toe of the foot.
5	**Anterior**	The "front" of the body	The sternum is on the anterior side of the body.
6	**Posterior**	The "back" of the body	The heel bone is on the posterior side of the foot.
7	**Proximal**	The part of a structure or organ located nearest to the point of origin (often the central axis of the body).	The elbow is proximal to the wrist.
8	**Distal**	The part of a structure or organ that is located farthest from the point of origin (often the central axis of the body).	The ankle is distal to the knee cap.

SUPERFICIAL BODY TERMINOLOGY

The following table lists a few select superficial body terms that will be used in this course on a regular basis. The best way to study these areas would be to examine the figures in the textbook to find the areas and then find the same areas on your own body. Then, practice verbalizing those terms and describing their location compared to another area using the terminology from the previous page. Keep in mind, there might be terms in this table that are not in the textbook.

Superficial Body Terms

	Head and Neck		Eyes	Ears
1	Frons	Occipital	Palpebra (eyelid)	Pinna
2	Glabella	Temporal	Palpebral fissure	Helix
3	Nasion	Zygomatic	Lateral commissure	Antihelix
4	Nasus	Otic	Medial commissure	Antitragus
5	Ala of the nose	Cervical	Pupil	Tragus
6	Nasolabial sulcus	Ocular	Sclera	Intertragic notch
7	Philtrum	Buccal	Iris	Ear lobe
8	Vermilion border			Triangular fossa
9	Oris			Crus
10	Mentis			Cymba
11				Scapha

SUPERFICIAL BODY TERMINOLOGY

The following table continues the list of select superficial body terms of the torso. Again, the best way to study these areas would be to examine the figures in the textbook to find the areas and then find the same areas on your own body. Again, practice verbalizing those terms and describing their location compared to another area using the terminology from previous pages. Again, keep in mind, there might be terms in this table that are not in the textbook.

Superficial Body Terms (continued)

		Torso	
		Anterior	**Posterior**
1		Axilla	Upper back (dorsum)
2		Thoracic	Lumbar
3		Mamma	Gluteal region
4		Abdomen	Gluteal fold
5		Umbilicus	Gluteal cleft
6		Pelvis	
7		Inguinal	

Superficial Body Terminology

The following table continues the list of select superficial body terms of the arms and legs. You will notice that sometimes there are two or three terms to describe the same body region. Some of the terms are Latin nouns and some are Latin adjectives. As long as the terms are descriptive and are not layman's terms, they are accurate. Again, practice verbalizing the terms while finding them on your own body.

Superficial Body Terms (continued)

	Arms	Legs
1	Brachium (brachial)	Iliac
2	Antecubital (antecubitis)	Femoral
3	Antebrachium (antebrachial)	Patella
4	Carpals (carpus)	Crus (entire lower leg)
5	Pollex	Tarsals
6	Cubital (olecranon)	Hallux
7		Popliteal (popliteus)
8		Sura (posterior lower leg only)
9		Calcaneal

SUPERFICIAL BODY TERMINOLOGY (PALPATION)

The following table lists a few select superficial body areas that you can feel on your own body. Many of these terms will be used again when we discuss the skeletal bones in later chapters.

Superficial Body Areas That You Can Feel (palpate)

	Upper Body	Lower Body
1	Nasal	Iliac
2	Zygomatic	Greater trochanter
3	Angle of the mandible	Patella
4	Mandible	Lateral epicondyle of the femur
5	Clavicle	Medial epicondyle of the femur
6	Medial border of the scapula	Tibial tuberosity
7	Spine of the scapula	Medial malleolus
8	Lateral epicondyle of the humerus	Lateral malleolus
9	Medial epicondyle of the humerus	Calcaneus
10	Olecranon	

BODY CAVITIES

Anatomists have subdivided the body into various cavities to assist in the study and understanding of the complexities of the body. The following table organizes the discussion of the body cavities.

Body Cavities

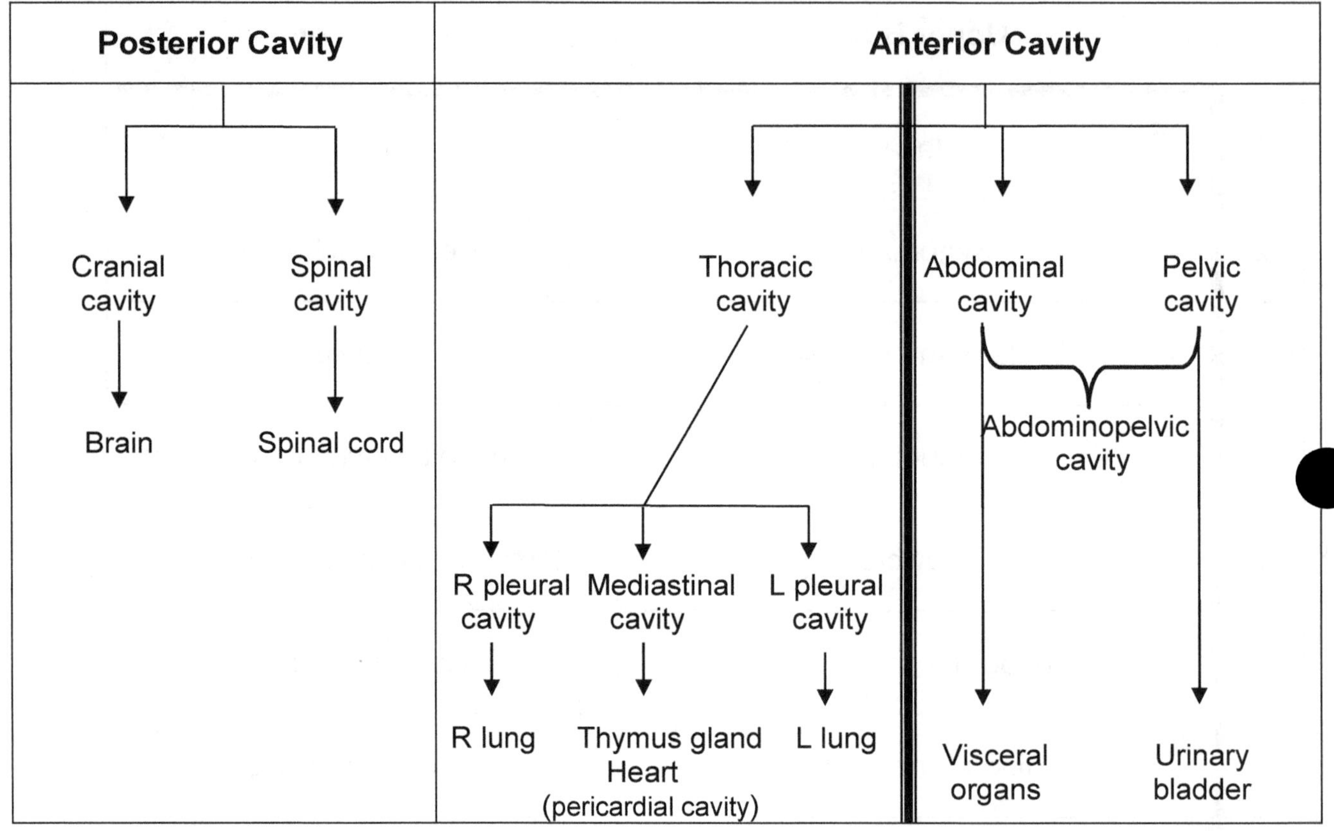

The diaphragm muscle creates a physical separation between the thoracic cavity and the abdominal cavity. There is not a physical separation between the abdominal cavity and the pelvic cavity. Therefore, the abdominal cavity and pelvic cavity are combined to form the **abdominopelvic cavity**. The dark line in the table represents the diaphragm muscle.

QUADRANTS AND ABDOMINOPELVIC REGIONS

There are numerous organs in the abdominopelvic cavity. In order to simplify the study of all these organs, anatomists have further subdivided the abdominopelvic cavity into four quadrants. Then, anatomists have subdivided the abdominopelvic cavity into even more detailed areas consisting of nine abdominopelvic regions. The following table below lists the quadrants and abdominopelvic regions and a few select organs or parts of organs within those areas.

Quadrants and Abdominopelvic Regions

Quadrants	Select Organs	Abdominopelvic Regions	Select Organs
Right upper quadrant	Liver, gallbladder, and transverse colon	**Epigastric**	Left lobe of liver
		Umbilical	Most of the small intestine
Left upper quadrant	Stomach, spleen, and transverse colon	**Hypogastric**	Ileum of small intestine and urinary bladder
		Right hypochondriac	Right lobe of liver and fundus of the liver
Right lower quadrant	Cecum, beginning ascending colon, and appendix	**Left hypochondriac**	Fundus of the stomach and spleen
		Right lumbar	Ascending colon
Left lower quadrant	Descending colon and sigmoid colon	**Left lumbar**	Descending colon
		Right inguinal	Cecum
		Left inguinal	Sigmoid colon

DISSECTIONAL CUTS (PLANES OF DISSECTION)

When an autopsy is performed, many times various tissues of the body need to be dissected. The tissue being cut needs to be described very precisely so that others looking at the autopsy report can understand it fully. In other words, the pathologist doing the autopsy cannot simply say, "I am cutting this piece of tissue in half." The following below identifies a few select dissectional cuts.

Dissectional Cuts

Dissectional Cut (Dissectional Plane)	Description
Frontal	Separating the anterior part of the tissue or organ from the posterior part
Sagittal*	Separating the right part of the tissue or organ from the left part
Transverse	Separating the superior part of the tissue or organ from the inferior part
Oblique	Making a dissectional cut at an angle across the tissue or organ

*Sagittal can be further divided into **parasagittal** (divided into unequal right and left regions) and **midsagittal** (divided into equal right and left regions).

ADDITIONAL TERMS

The following table lists a few select terms that will be used throughout the course of your anatomy study.

Additional Terms

	Term	Description
1	**Superficial**	On the surface or near the surface of the body.
2	**Deep**	Deeper into the body. Farthest away from the superficial. Moving towards the interior of the body.
3	**Intermediate**	Tissue that is located somewhere between two other pieces of tissue (such as between a superficial tissue and a deep tissue).
4	**Bilateral**	Found on both sides of the body on the same structure (e.g., a disorder found in both kidneys)
5	**Unilateral**	Found on one side of the body (e.g., a disorder found only in one kidney)
6	**Ipsilateral**	Found on the same side of the body but not the same structure (e.g., a disorder found on the left arm and the left leg)
7	**Contralateral**	Found on the opposite side of the body but not on the same structure (e.g., a disorder found on the left arm and the right leg)

Additional Terms (continued)

	Term	Description
8	**Flex** **(flexion)**	Decrease the angle at the joint between two bones.
9	**Extend** **(extension)**	Increase the angle at the joint between two bones.
10	**Abduct** **(abduction)**	To take away from the body or move away from the midline. (to abduct your arm means to move your arm laterally).
11	**Adduct** **(adduction)**	To add back to the body or move toward the midline. (to adduct your arm means to move your arm from a lateral position to a medial position).
12	**Supinate** **(supination)**	Palms are anterior; the palms will be "facing up" when the arm is bent at a 90° angle (you can hold a cup of soup).
13	**Pronate** **(pronation)**	Palms are posterior (the palms will be "facing downward" when the arm is bent at a 90° angle).

Below is some additional information regarding the muscles of the head and neck region. Your instructor may add to this list.

1. The word "anatomy" is derived from the Greek word "anatome," which means "to cut."

2. The word "autopsy" is Greek, which means "to see for oneself."

3. The umbilical is medial and inferior to the nipple region.

4. The patella region is anterior to the popliteal region.

5. The hypochondriac regions are immediately lateral to the epigastric region.

6. The term "chondriac" refers to cartilage. The word "hypo" refers to below or under an area. The right and left hypochondriac are regions that are below and under a lot of cartilage associated with the ribs.

7. The mediastinal cavity is the cavity that is between the pleural cavities.

8. A midsagittal dissection is a cut that equally divides the right side of a piece of tissue from the left side of the tissue.

9. A parasagittal dissection is a cut that does not equally divide the tissue when it is dissected.

10. The stomach is located just a bit to the left of the midline of the body and the spleen is on the left lateral edge of the stomach.

11. Spelling is important. There is a difference between ilium and ileum and between coracoid and coronoid.

Chapter 2:   Cells and Tissues

There are over 75 trillion cells in the human body. Anatomists have categorized the cells to make it easier to study and understand their functions. All of the cells of the human body have been placed into groups of tissue categories. There are four main types of tissues that make up the human body.

	Tissue Type	Characteristic
1	Epithelial tissue	The cells that belong in this category make up the inside or outside lining of an organ.
2	Muscular tissue	The cells that belong in this category have the ability to contract and relax.
3	Neural tissue	The cells that belong in this category have the ability to transmit an impulse or are involved in providing protection for the cells that transmit impulses.
4	Connective tissue	The cells that belong in this category have a matrix of some sort. The cells are embedded in the matrix. This tissue type serves to connect, bind, surround, or enclose various structures. Some of the cells in this tissue category do not actually connect anything.

Study the following four items while referring to the following table.

1. The cell's issue type.
2. Appearance of the cell.
3. Function of the cell.
4. Sample location of the cell in the body.

Epithelial Tissue	
Squamous cells	In deeper tissue, these cells appear round. As you approach the surface of the tissue, the cells become flattened. These cells provide physical protection. Cells can be found making up the inside lining of the mouth and the outside lining of the skin.
Cuboid cells	These cells appear to be cube-shaped. These cells secrete and absorb material. Cells can be found making up the lining of the urinary tubes and some glands.
Columnar cells	These cells appear to be longer than they are wide. These cells secrete and absorb material. Cells can be found making up the lining of the trachea and the small intestine.

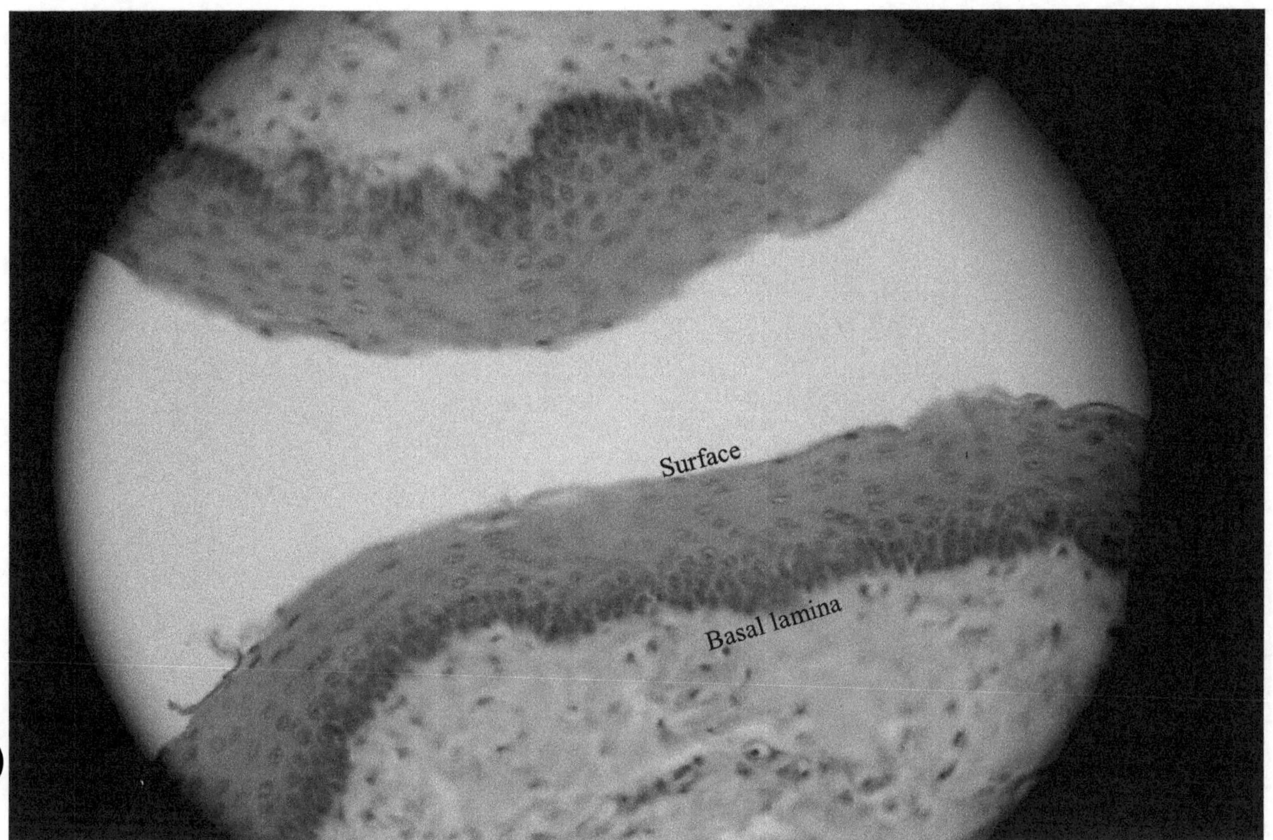

Notice: The cells are sort-of roundish near the **basal lamina** area. As you migrate closer to the surface area, the cells begin to flatten. The nucleus appears to be "squished."

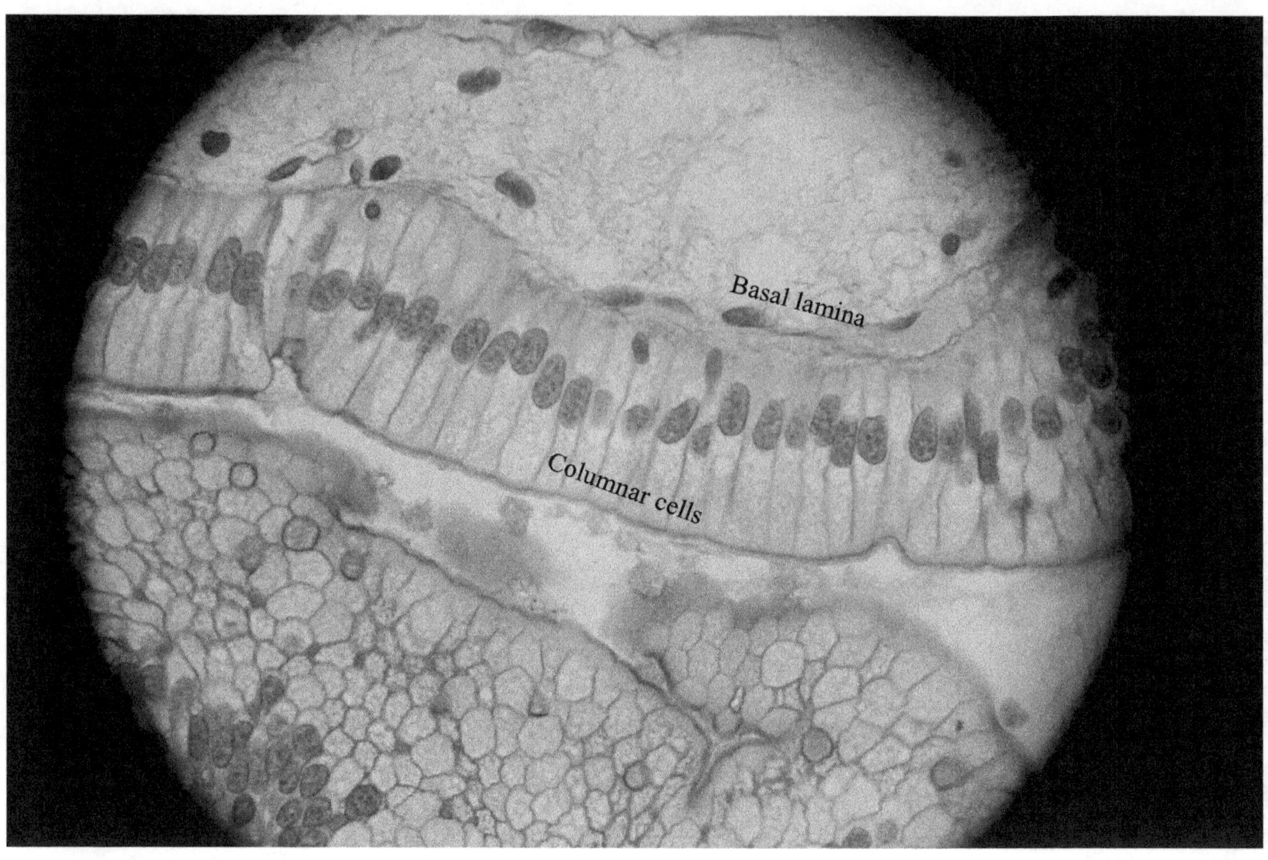

Notice: The cells appear to be longer than they are wide.

These are simple columnar cells. Notice how the nuclei appear to be fairly "inline" from cell to cell.

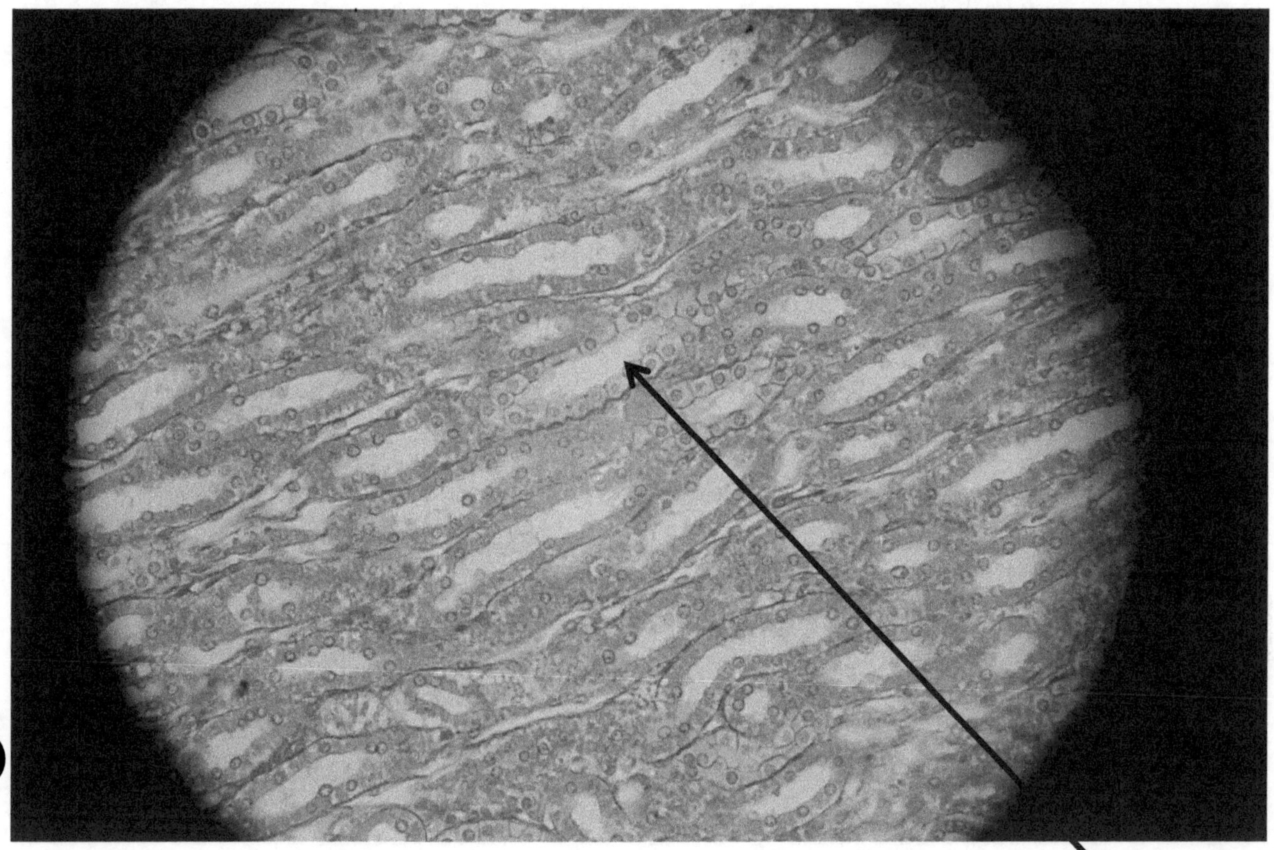

Notice: The cuboid cells form the lining of a tube. The inside of the tube is the **lumen**.

Study the following four items while referring to the following table.

1. The cell's tissue type.
2. Appearance of the cell.
3. Function of the cell.
4. Sample location of the cell in the body.

Muscular Tissue	
Skeletal muscle cells	When viewed under a microscope, these cells appear to be striped (striated). These cells provide voluntary contraction. Cells can be found making up the arm and leg muscles.
Smooth muscle cells	These cells appear to have pointed ends (spindle-shaped). The nucleus appears flattened with pointed ends as well. These cells provide involuntary contraction. Cells can be found making up sphincter muscles, myometrium, and the blood vessels.
Cardiac muscle cells	These cells are associated with intercalated discs. These cells provide rhythmic or pulsating contractions. Cells are found only in the myocardium of the heart.

SKELETAL MUSCLE CELLS

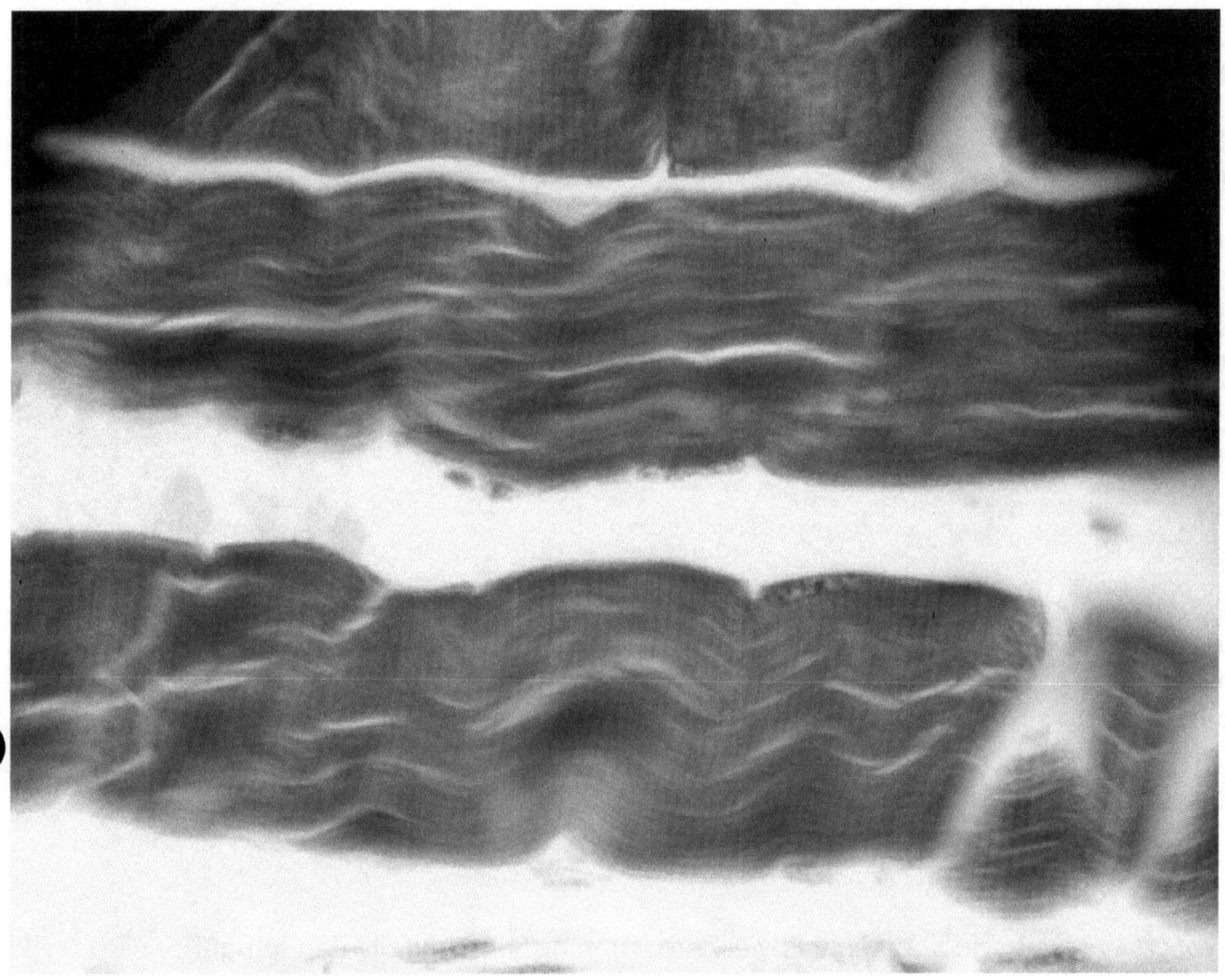

Notice: The muscle fibers in this view are "running" horizontally (left to right).

The striations are perpendicular.

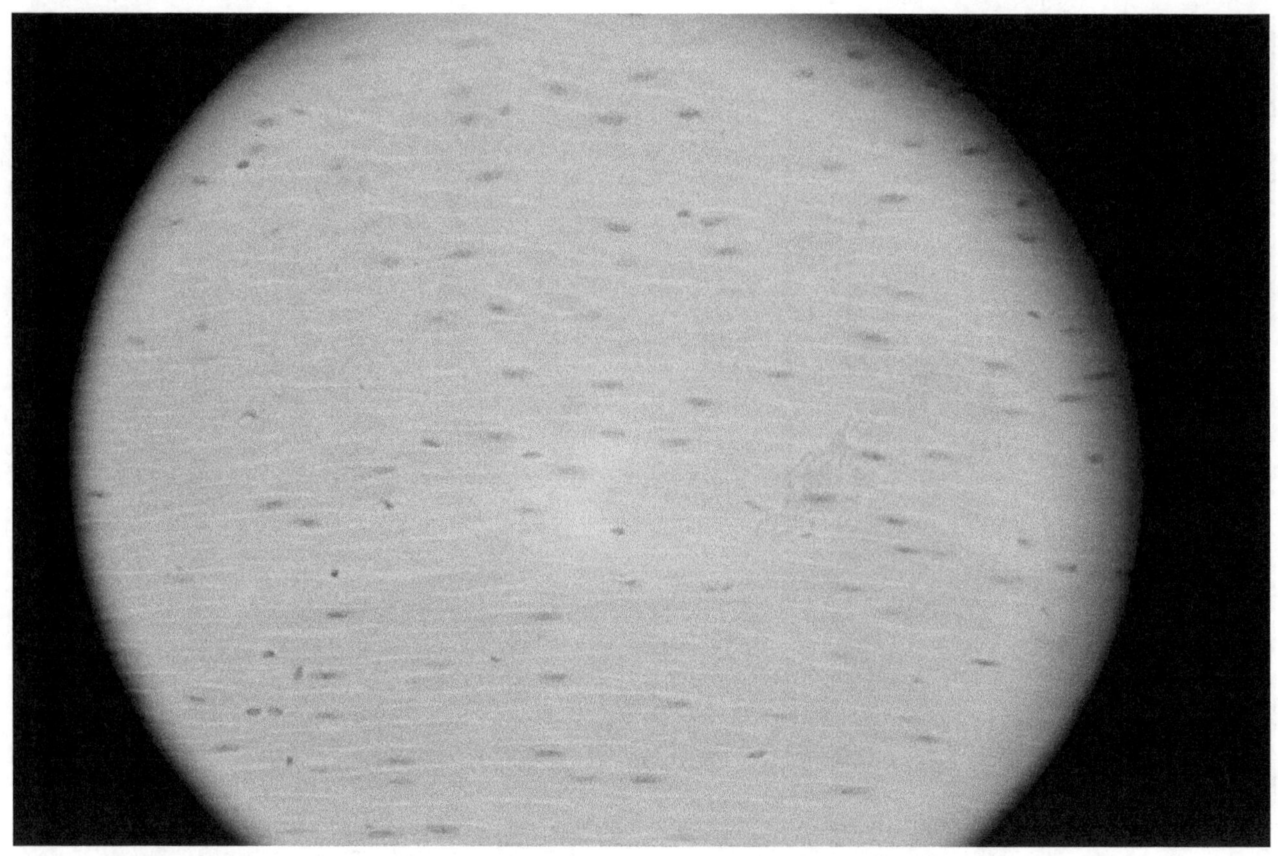

Notice: The muscle fibers in this view are "running" horizontally (left to right).

It is very difficult to see the individual cells. The individual cells have tapered ends.

The nucleus within each fiber appears to have tapered ends.

This is called smooth muscle because it lacks striations.

CARDIAC MUSCLE CELLS

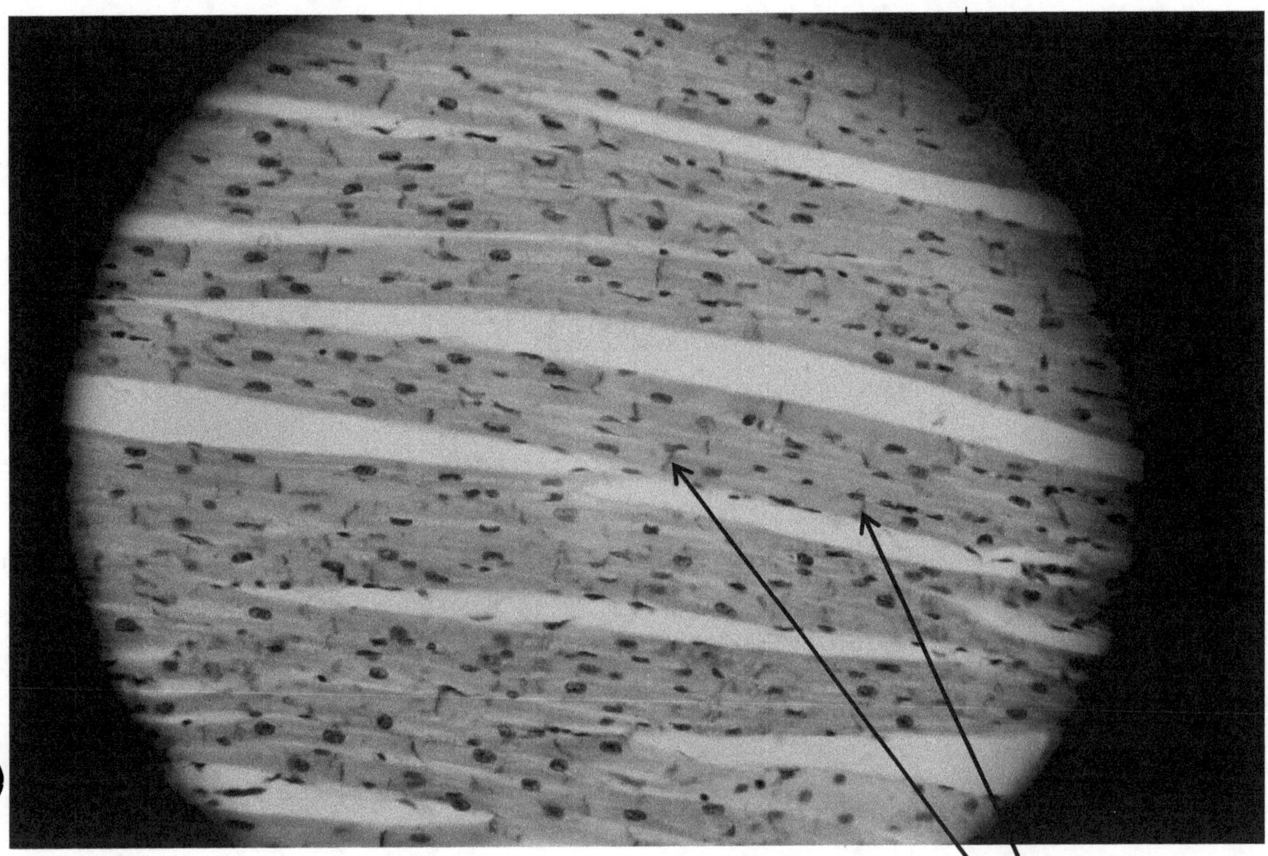

Notice: The muscle fibers are "running" horizontally (left to right).

The main characteristic of cardiac cells is the presence of **<u>intercalated discs</u>**.

These disks appear as dark bands, which are intermittent bands that are

perpendicular to the muscle fiber.

NEURAL TISSUE

Study the following four items while referring to the following table.

1. The cell's tissue type.
2. Appearance of the cell.
3. Function of the cell.
4. Sample location of the cell in the body.

Neural Tissue	
Neurons	These cells have extensions branching off the soma. These cells conduct impulses. Cells can be found making up the brain tissue.
Glial cells	These cells take on a variety of shapes. These cells provide protection for the neurons. Cells can be found surrounding the axon of the neuron or in close proximity to the neuron.

Neural Cells (Neuron and Glial Cells)

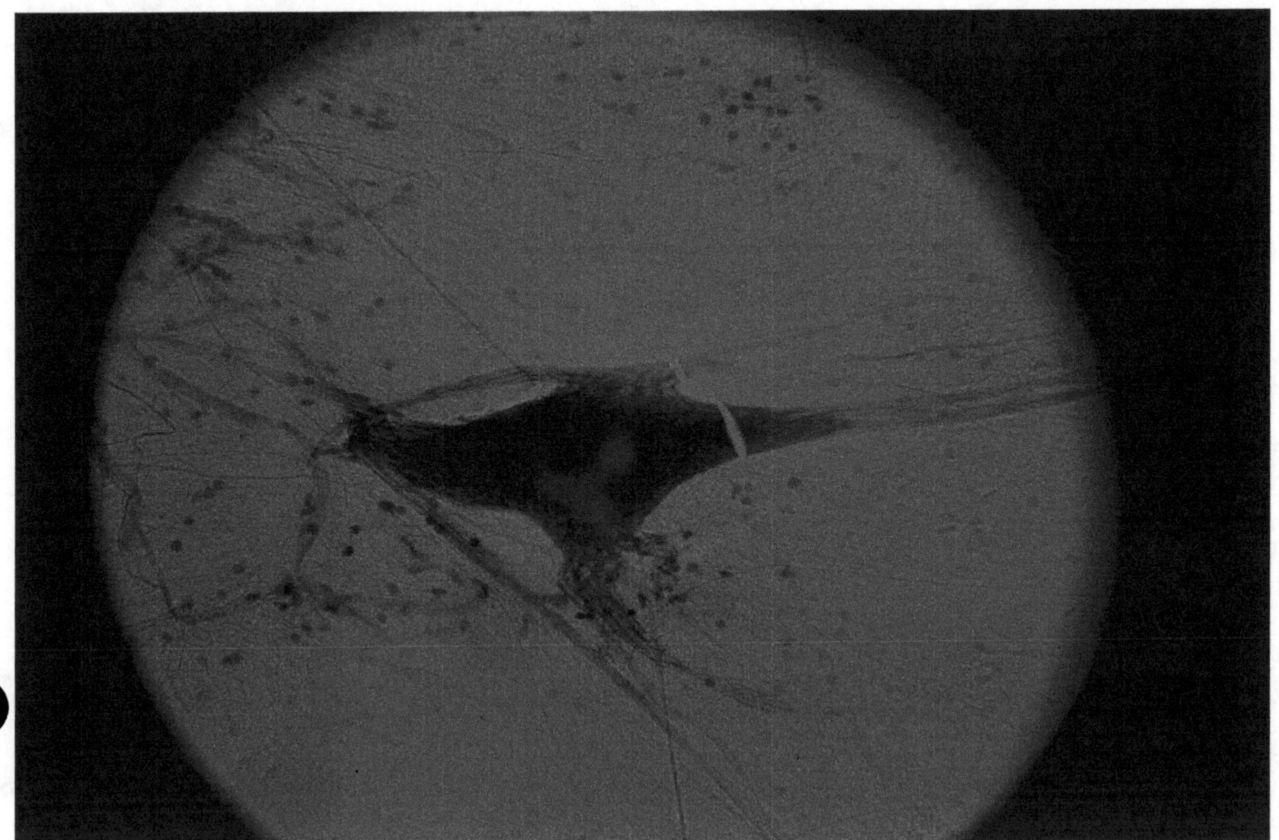

Notice: A neuron consists of a soma, dendrite, and axon. The branches off the soma are the dendrites and axon. The shorter branches off the soma are the dendrites and the longer branches are axons. Some neurons have only one axon.

The glial cells are scattered throughout this image. In this image, they appear as small dots.

Study the following five items while referring to the following tables.

1. The cell's tissue type.
2. Appearance of the cell.
3. Function of the cell.
4. Sample location of the cell in the body.
5. Type of matrix involved (see the following table).

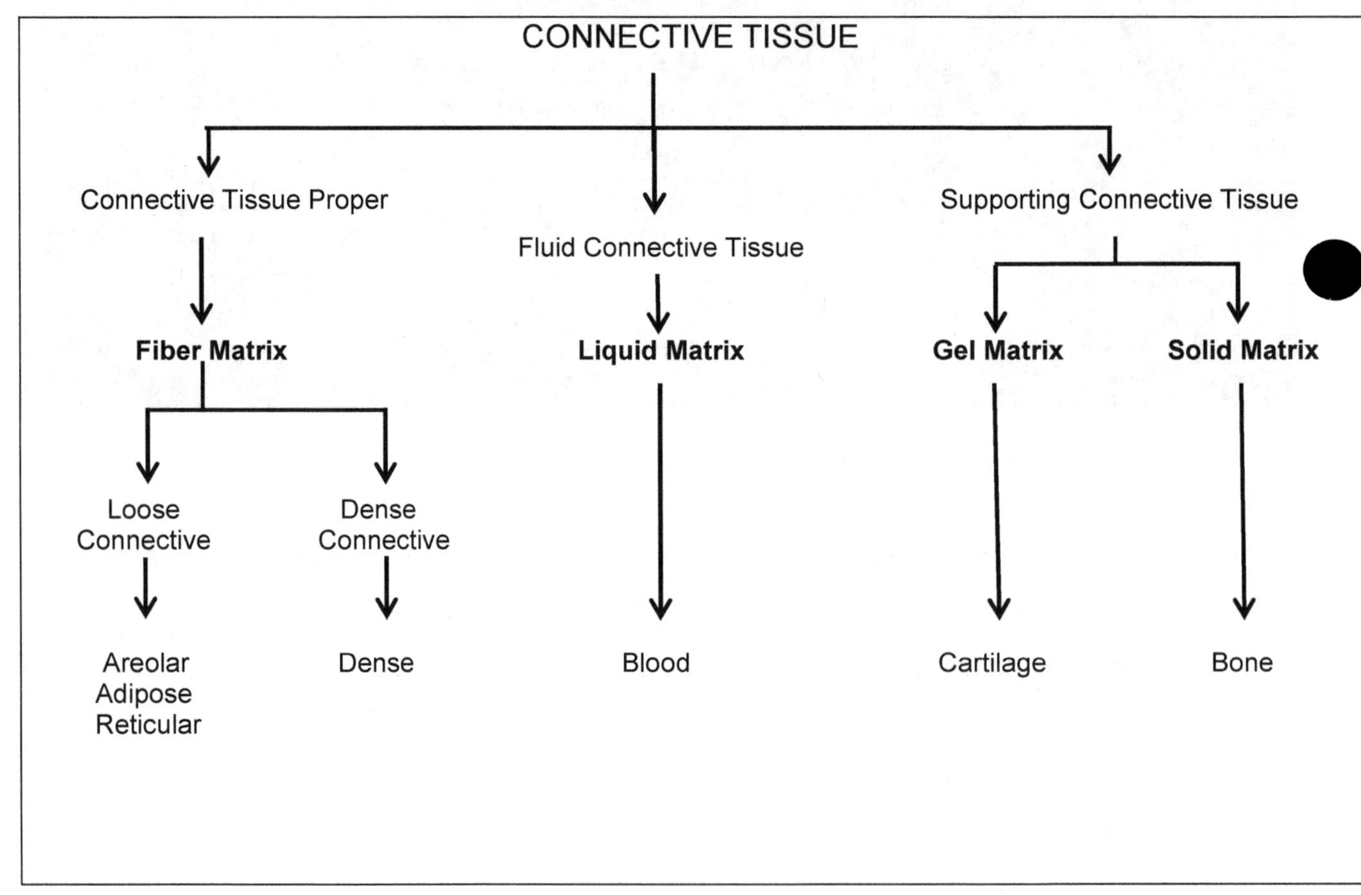

Adipose tissue (adipocytes)	These cells generally appear round and have the appearance that they are empty. These cells provide: 1. insulation for organs of the body 2. protection and cushion 3. stored energy (li[ids) Cells can be found surrounding body organs.
Areolar tissue (areolar cells)	These cells (fibrocytes) are small and have numerous, thin hair-like fibers coursing between the cells. These fibers provide a physical attachment of the skin to muscle. Cells are located between the skin and muscle.
Reticular tissue	These are small cells that have short, thick fibers coursing between them. These cells make up the framework of many organs. Cells make up the liver, spleen, appendix, tonsils, and thymus gland (for example)
Dense tissue	These cells appear to be packed tightly together to form strong fibrous strands of material. These cells form strong connections. Cells are found associated with tendons, ligaments, and aponeuroses.

Areolar Tissue (Cells)

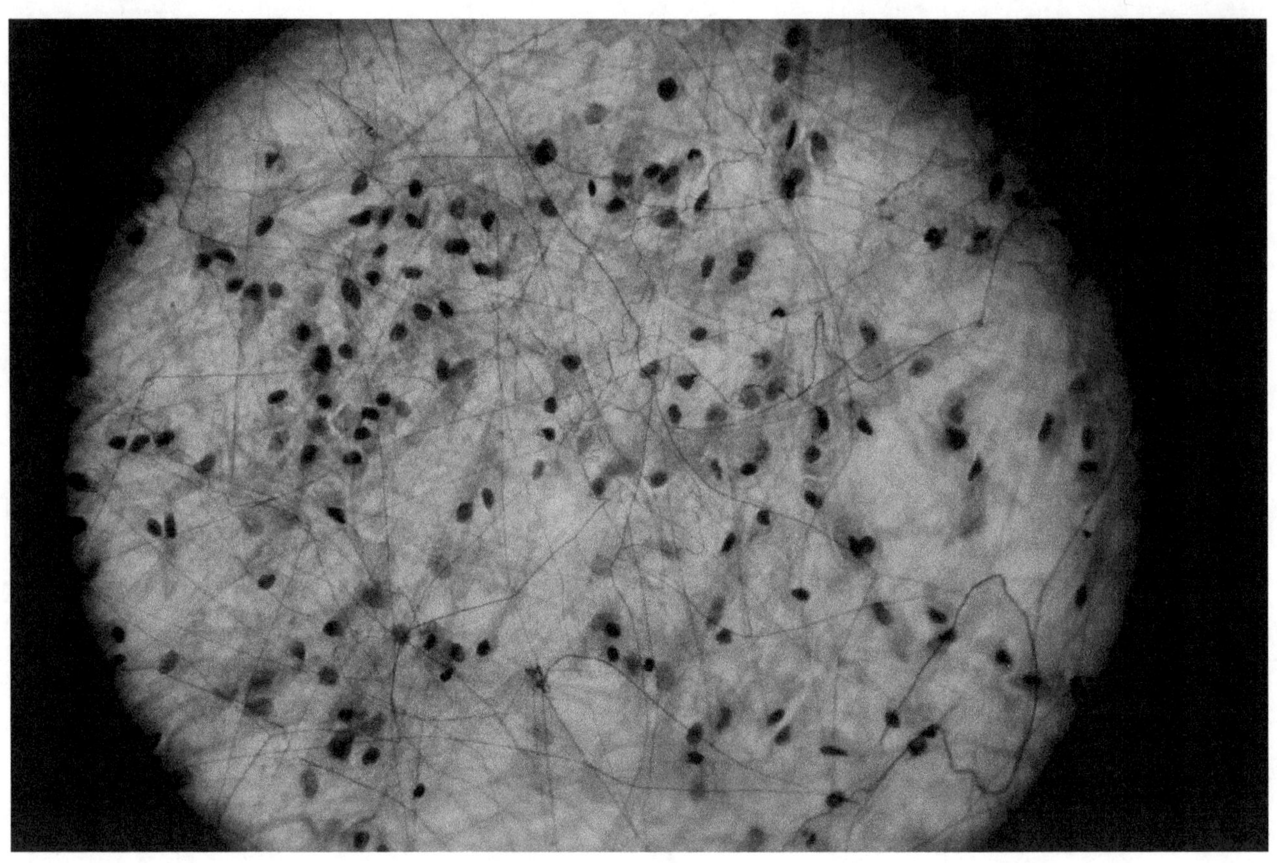

Notice: Areolar tissue consists of fibrocytes, which produce numerous fibers that are long and thin, giving the tissue its "hair-like" appearance.

There is a lot of space between the fibers, giving the tissue its loose characteristic and thus the tissue does not provide very strong attachment.

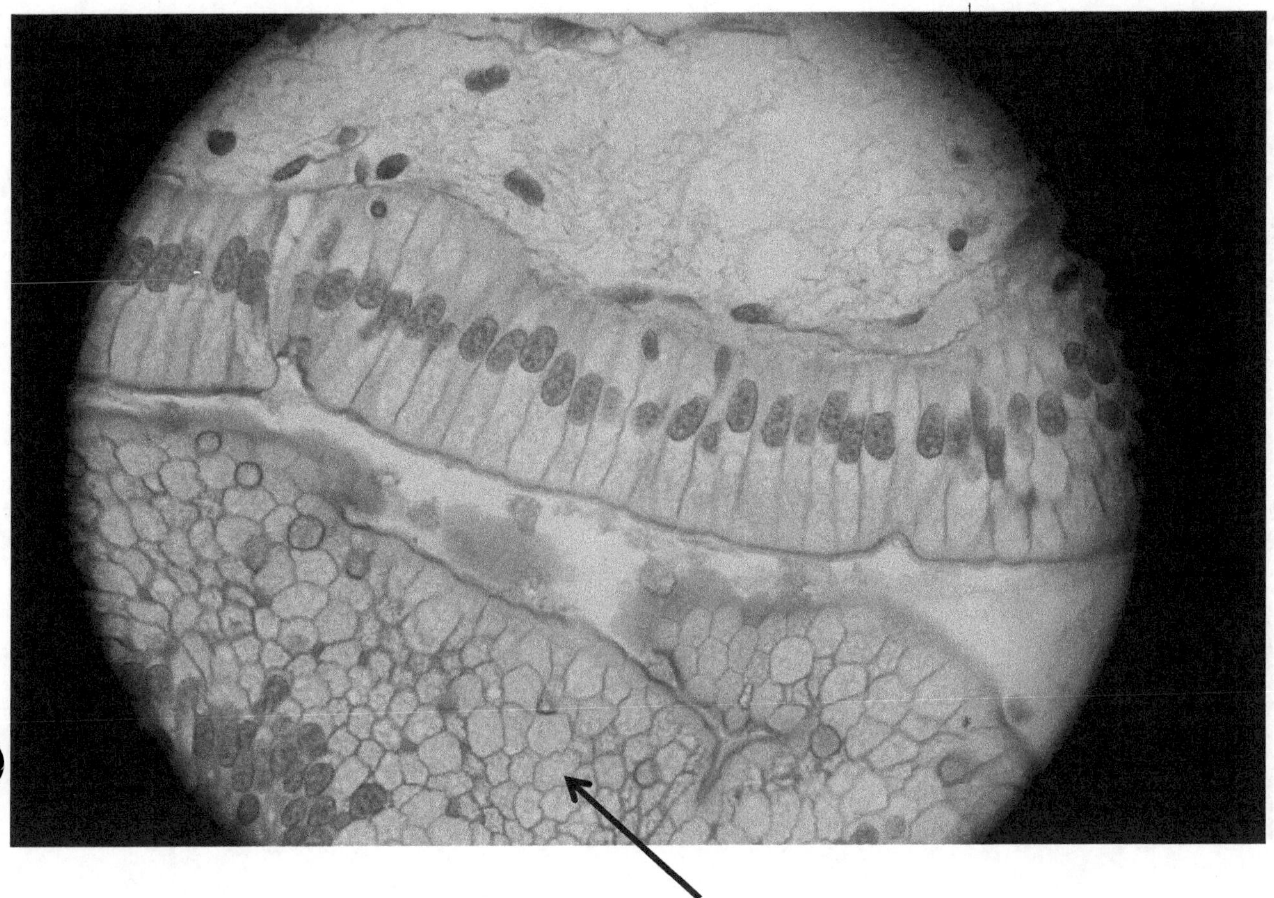

Notice: The top portion of this view consists of columnar cells. The lower portion
consists of adipocytes (arrow).

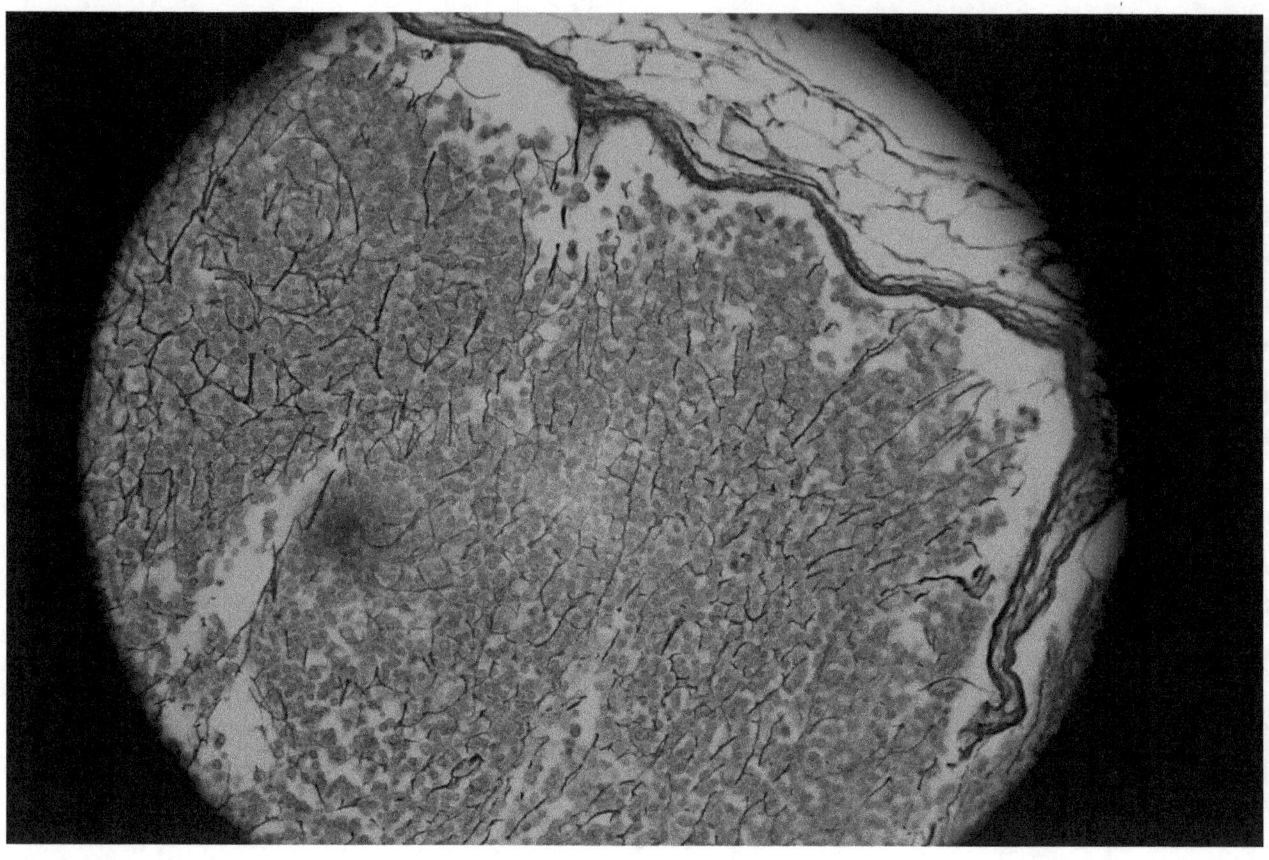

Notice: The round cells are fibroblast cells.

The matrix is the short, thick, irregular, dark fibers.

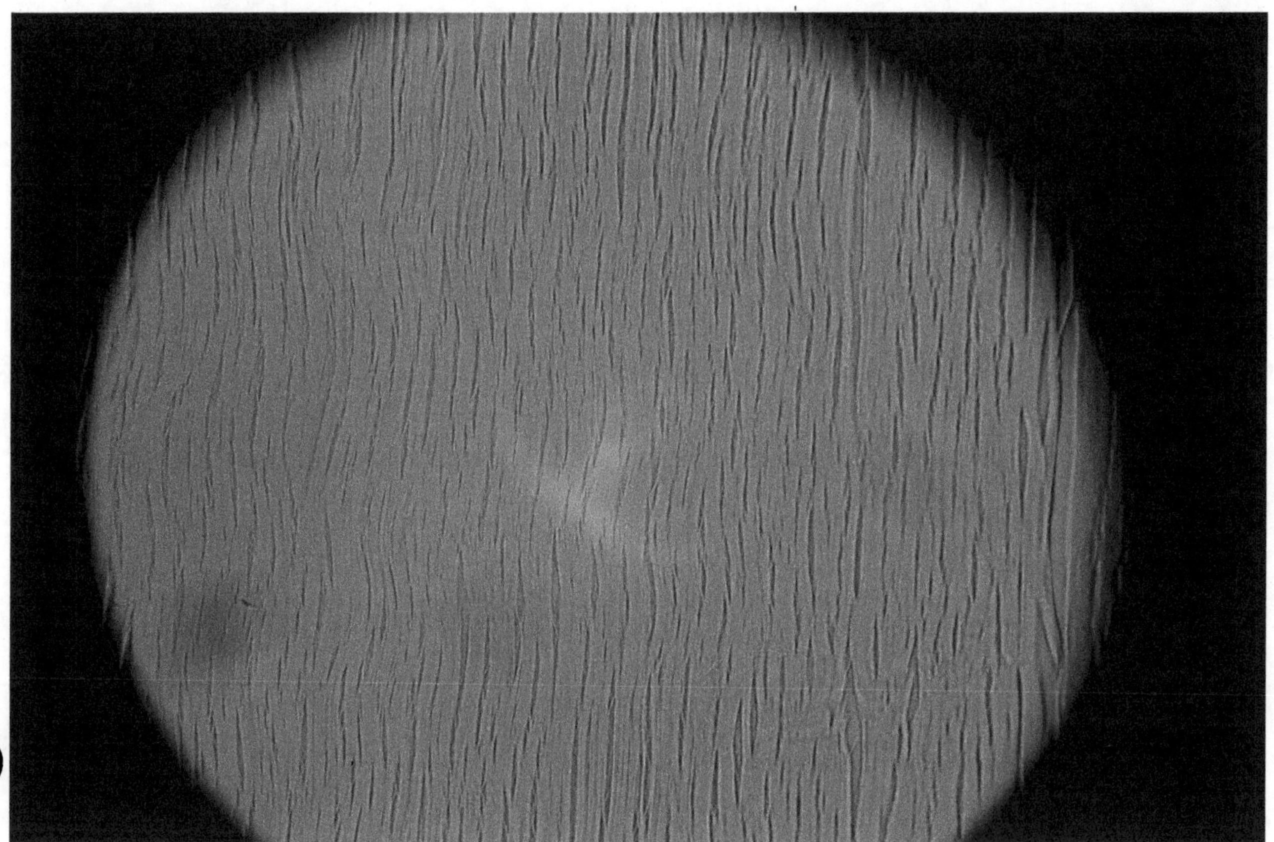

Notice: The dense fibers are "running" vertically (in this example).

You cannot see individual cells.

You can see the fiber matrix, which appears as dark bands also "running" vertically.

CONNECTIVE TISSUE WITH A LIQUID MATRIX

Blood tissue (blood cells)	These cells are small and have plasma flowing between them. Refer to the "Additional Information" section to see the functions. Cells are found in the circulatory system.

CONNECTIVE TISSUE WITH A SOLID MATRIX

Bone tissue (osteocytes)	The osteocytes form concentric rings around a central canal. These cells provide strength. Cells are found associated with our skeleton.

CONNECTIVE TISSUE WITH A GEL MATRIX

Cartilage tissue (chondrocytes)	These cells appear to have a lot of white area around them. These cells provide flexibility. Cells are found within the joints and flexible parts of the helix of the ear and the ala of the nose.

BLOOD CELLS

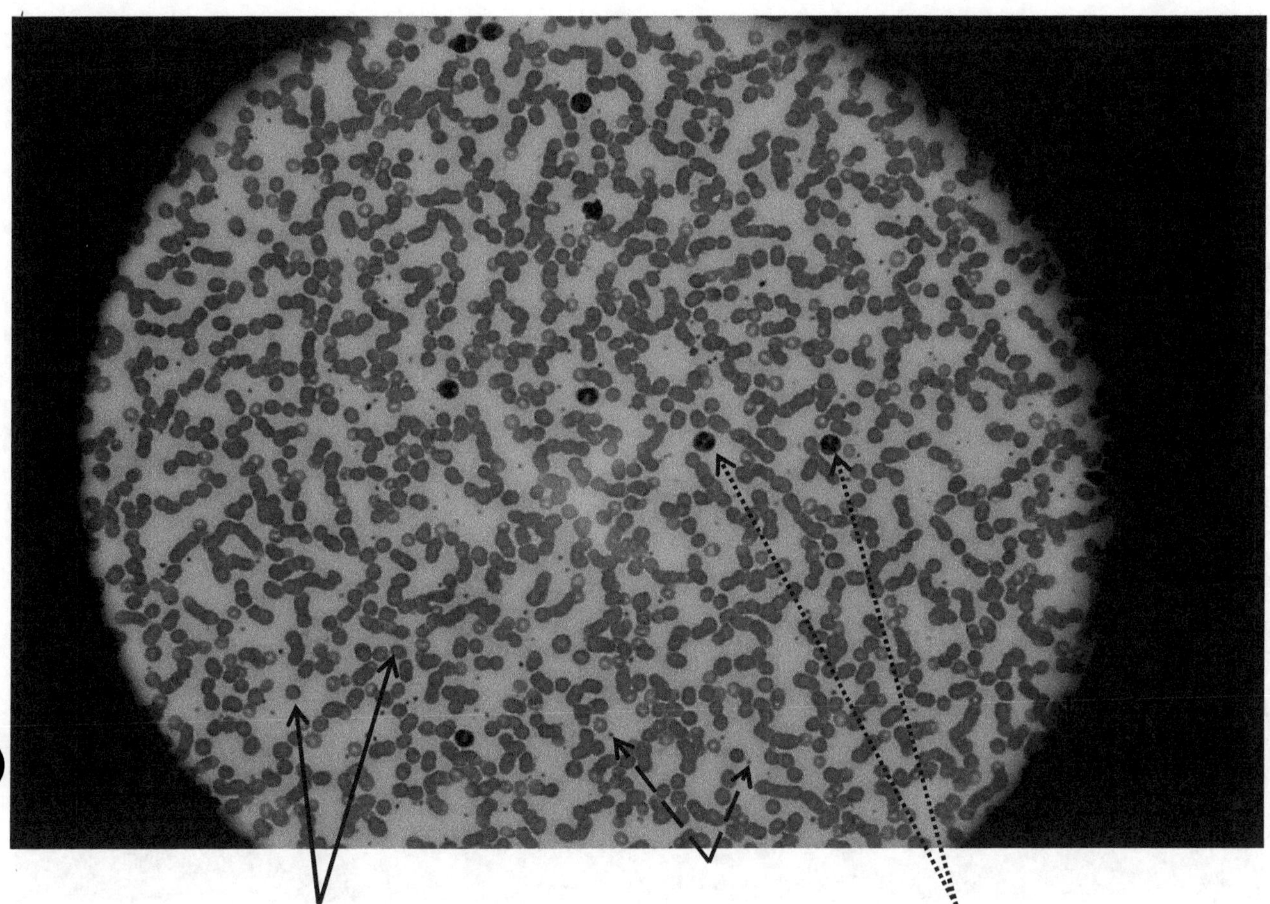

Notice: There are three main cellular components that make up blood.

Red blood cells (**erythrocytes**) — solid arrow

White blood cells (**leukocytes**) — dotted arrow

Platelets (**thrombocytes**) — dashed arrow

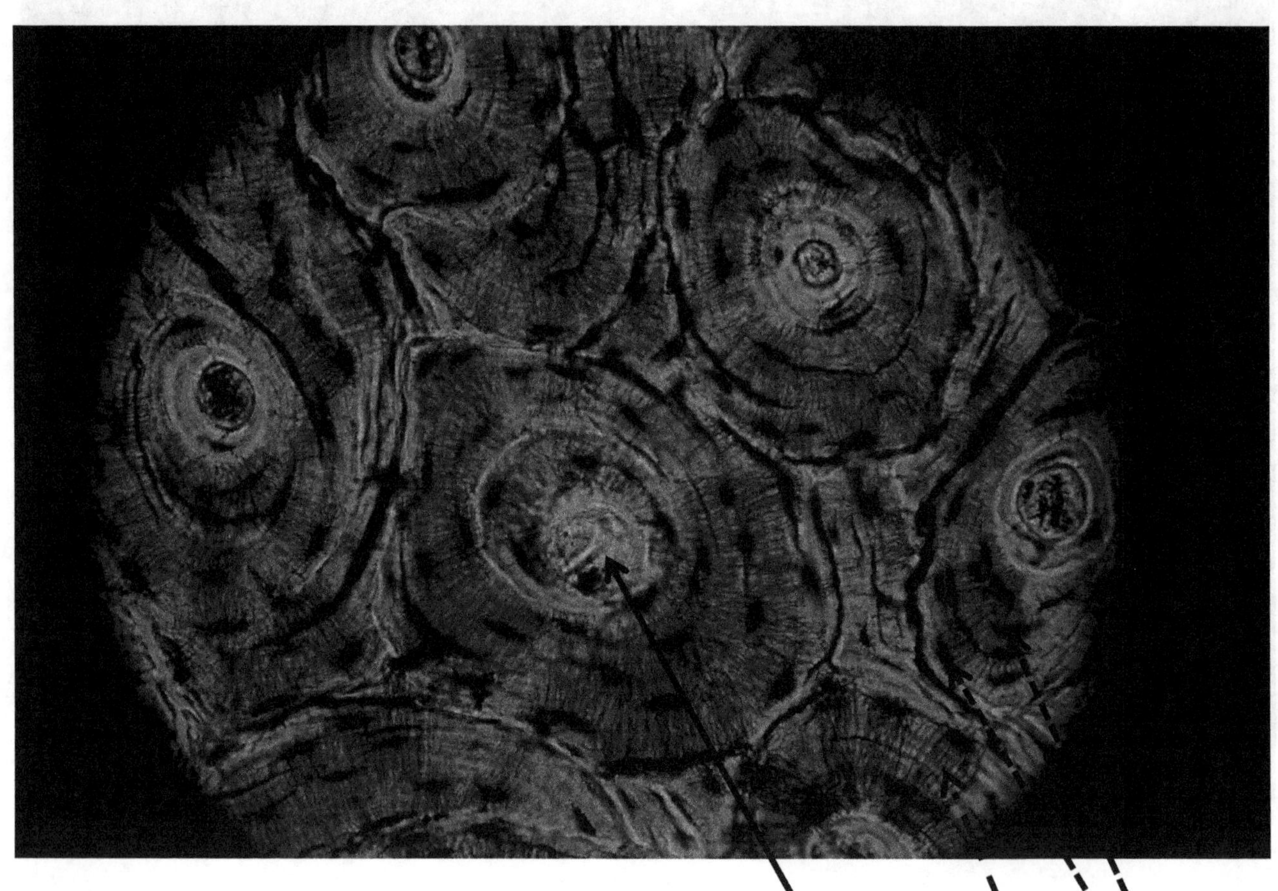

Notice: Bone tissue is made of **osteons**.

Each osteon consists of:

Central canal ⟶

Osteocytes ----➤

Lacuna (osteocytes are sitting in the **lacuna**)

Canaliculi — · —➤

Lamellae   (canaliculi pass through the lamellae)

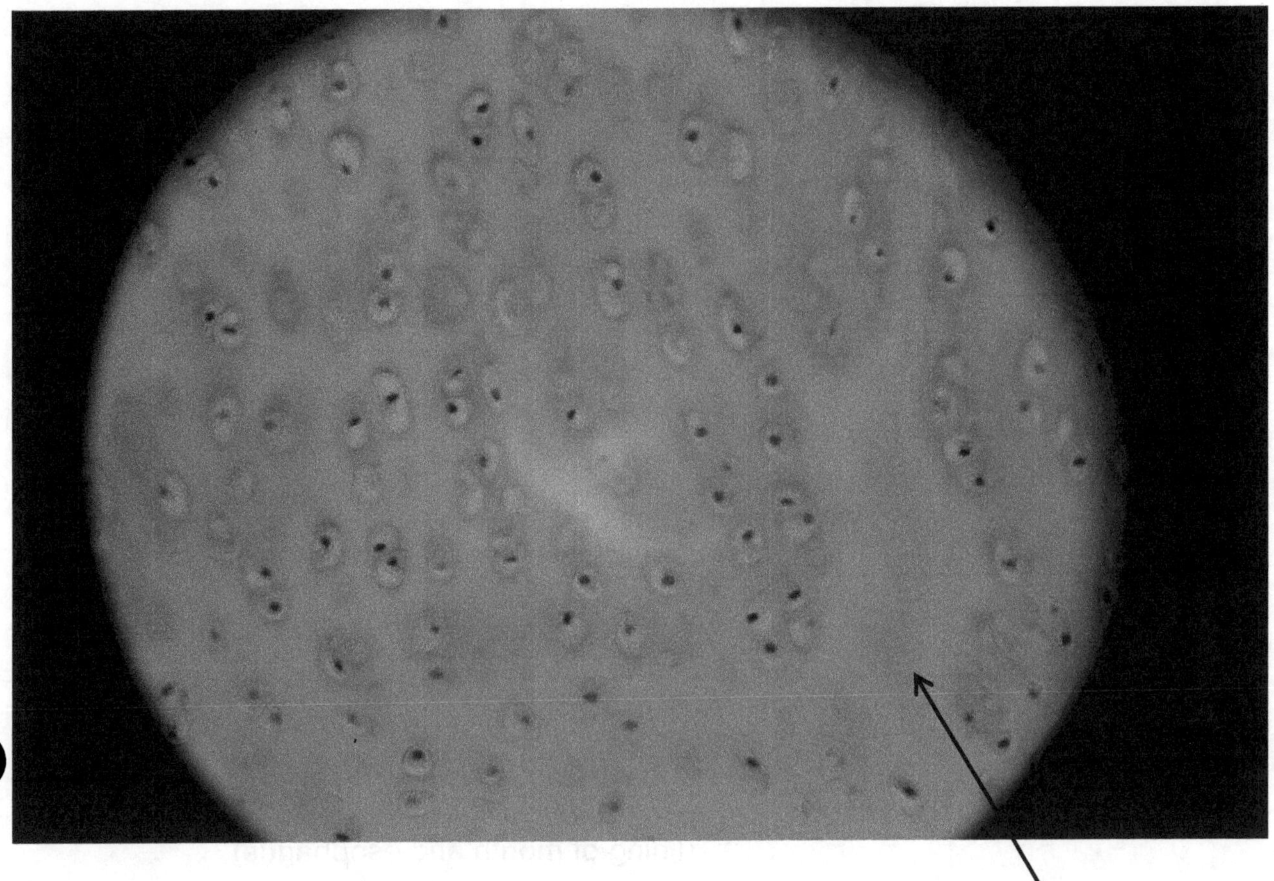

Notice: Chondrocytes sit in a depression called a **lacuna**.

Each lacuna is larger than the individual cartilage cell (hence the white space around the cartilage cell).

The flexibility of cartilage is due to its gel matrix.

Additional Epithelial Cell Types ( ) = location	
Simple epithelial tissue	Simple squamous. 　　Single layer of squamous cells. 　　　　　　(alveoli and capillary walls) Simple cuboidal. 　　Single layer of cuboid cells. 　　　　　　(glands and kidney tubes) Simple columnar. 　　Single layer of columnar cells. 　　　The nuclei are pretty much in a row along the basement membrane. 　　　　　　(uterine tubes and respiratory tract)
Stratified epithelial tissue	Stratified squamous. 　　Several layers of squamous cells. The apical cells are flat shaped. 　　　　　　(lining of mouth and esophagus) Stratified cuboidal. 　　Several layers of cuboidal cells. The apical cells are cube-shaped. 　　　　　　(rare – found in parts of the male urethra) Stratified columnar. 　　Several layers of columnar cells. The apical cells are columnar-shaped. 　　　　　　(rare – found in parts of the male urethra)

MORE EPITHELIAL CELL TYPES (CONTINUED)

Additional Epithelial Cell Types ( ) = location	
Pseudostratified epithelial tissue	Pseudostratified columnar. One layer of cells but of varying heights. The nuclei are also at different heights within each columnar cell. These cells can be ciliated or non-ciliated. (trachea -- ciliated) (ductus deferens -- non ciliated)
Transitional epithelial tissue	Tissue consists of cells that have a variety of shapes. This tissue is extremely stretchable-- (lines the urinary bladder)

Below is some additional information regarding the muscles of the head and neck region. Your instructor may add to this list.

1. Some columnar cells have cilia at their apical ends.

2. Since muscle cells are so long, they are sometimes referred to as muscle fibers. Do not confuse muscle fibers with the fiber matrix material.

3. Neurons are made of an axon, a soma, and a dendrite. The soma is the cell body and consists of the nucleus.

4. There are several types of glial cells. Some protect the nerves of the central nervous system while others protect the peripheral nervous system.

    a. Glial cells of the central nervous system

        i. **Astrocytes**: These cells form connections between neurons and blood vessels. These cells help to create the blood-brain barrier.

        ii. **Microglia**: These cells defend against pathogens.

        iii. **Oligodendrocytes**: These cells myelinate the central nervous system axons.

    b. Glial cells of the peripheral nervous sytem

        i. **Satellite** cells protect the somas.

        ii. **Neurolemmocytes** myelinate the peripheral nervous system axons.

5. There are three main cells that make up blood.

    a. **Erythrocytes** transport oxygen and carbon dioxide.

    b. **Leukocytes** provide our second line of defense. The skin is considered to be the first line of defense.

    c. **Platelets** are involved in blood clotting.

6. The solid portion of bone is made of five main components that comprise the main unit of bone called an **osteon**.

    a. **Osteocytes** are the individual bone cells.

    b. The **central canal** is the hollow portion in the center of the osteon. It consists of blood vessels.

    c. The **canaliculi** are small canals that transport nutrients from the blood vessels in the central canal to the individual osteocytes.

    d. The **lacuna** is a depression in the matrix in which the osteocytes reside.

    e. Bone is made of a solid matrix. The name for this matrix is **lamella**.

7. There are three main types of cellular material that compose the dense tissue category.

    a. **Tendons** connect muscle to bone.

    b. **Ligaments** connect bone to bone.

    c. **Aponeurosis** connects muscle to muscle.

8. Dense tissue heals slowly after injury (such as stretching or tearing a tendon or ligament). They heal slowly (if at all) because the tissue is avascular. It is avascular in order to have the strength that is required by tendons and ligaments. Other tissues of the body are vascular, so they heal much faster.

9. Cells are held together to make "sheets" of tissue by special connectors.

    a. **Desmosomes**: Small protein fibers that connect one cell with another.

    b. **Tight junctions**: Plasma protein that completely encircles the apical end of one cell with the apical end of another cell.

    c. **Gap junctions**: A bridge of proteins that forms a tunnel between one cell and another cell.

10. The base of cells is attached to the basal lamina and the apical end is the surface of the cell.

11. Almost all cells are nucleated. The erythrocytes are anucleated. The reason for this is studied in a physiology class. Skeletal muscle cells are typically multinucleated

12. Adipocytes are cells that are filled with molecules of fat. It is actually a misnomer to call them "fat cells."

13. **Hypertrophy** is an increase in cell size.
    Muscles increase protein filaments within the cells and the cells enlarge, thus giving the muscle a bulky appearance.

14. **Hyperplasia** is an increase in cell number.
    In early stages of pregnancy, the uterus increases in size due to hyperplasia. Then, it increases more due to hypertrophy.

15. **Metaplasia** is a change from one cell type to another cell type.
    In heavy smokers, the columnar cells of the trachea die and are replaced by squamous cells. Squamous cells provide protection against the harsh chemicals involved with smoking but do not have cilia to move mucus out of the trachea, hence, the development of the "smoker's cough."

Chapter 3: The Integumentary System

COMPONENTS OF THE INTEGUMENTARY SYSTEM

The **integumentary system** is composed of more than "just skin." It is composed of glands, nails, hair, and skin. An **organ** is defined as a group of tissues functioning together to perform various tasks. The "skin" is made of various tissues performing the task of providing protection from infection and injury. Therefore, the skin is an organ. It is the largest organ of the body. The following table identifies the structures of the integumentary system to be studied in this class.

	Integumentary component	Feature
1	**Skin**	The skin is composed of the epidermis and dermis. The epidermis is composed of four and sometimes five layers. The dermis is composed of two layers.
2	**Glands**	There are four major glands of the integumentary system. **Ceruminous glands** Located in the ear canal. Produce **cerumen** (ear wax). **Sebaceous glands** Located everywhere except the palms and soles. Produce **sebum**. **Apocrine glands** Located mostly around the nipple and inguinal region. Produce a special type of sweat that has an odor to it (**pheromones**). **Merocrine glands** Located everywhere. Produce sweat for cooling purposes.

	Integumentary component	Feature
3	**Nails**	A continuous growth of the epidermis. Provide minimal protection for the distal ends of the digits. Nail structures are mentioned in the "additional information" section.
4	**Hair**	Provides minimal protection for the skin.
5	**Epidermis**	Superficial layer of the integument. Consists of 4 (and in some areas 5) layers of tissue.
6	**Dermis**	Consists of 2 layers (papillary and reticular layer). This layer is deep to the epidermis. The papillary layer consists of the sebaceous glands and arrector pili muscles. The reticular layer consists of sweat glands (apocrine and merocrine glands).

LAYERS OF THE EPIDERMIS

The epidermis is made of four, and in some places five, different layers. The following table identifies the different layers of the epidermis and gives a brief description of each layer.

	Epidermis Layer	Feature
1	**Stratum corneum**	This is the most superficial layer of the epidermis. Made of dehydrated squamous cells.
2	**Stratum granulosum**	This is the next layer (deep to the stratum corneum). This layer consists of cells that produce a protein called **keratin**.
3	**Stratum spinosum**	This is the next layer (deep to the stratum granulosum). This layer has cells bound together by **desmosomes**.
4	**Stratum germinativum**	This is the deepest layer of the epidermis. This layer is also called the stratum basale. This layer forms the dermal papillae, thus creating the ridges we call fingerprints. This layer consists of melanocytes (discussed later). The cells in this layer have the ability to reproduce.
5	**Stratum lucidum**	When present, this layer is located between the stratum corneum and the stratum granulosum. When present, this skin is referred to as "thick skin." Located in callused areas.

LAYERS OF THE DERMIS

The dermis is made of two layers. The following table identities those two layers with a brief description of each layer.

	Dermis Layer	Feature
1	**Papillary layer**	This is the most superficial layer of the dermis. This layer is deep to the stratum germinativum. The main components of this layer are as follows: **Sebaceous glands** Glands that produce sebum. Sebum goes to the surface of the epidermis to lubricate the epidermis. **Arrector pili muscles** Arrector pili muscles are smooth muscles that extend from the shaft of the hair to the epidermis. Upon contraction, these muscles create "goose bumps." Each time a muscle (even tiny muscles like the arrector pili muscles) contract, they generate heat. Therefore, creating "goose bumps" is a way of generating heat for the body.
2	**Reticular layer**	This layer is deep to the papillary layer. This layer consists of sweat glands (apocrine and merocrine).

THE HYPODERMIS

While discussing the integumentary system, it is quite common to discuss the hypodermis at the same time. The hypodermis is technically not a part of the integumentary system. However, it is the tissue that is deep to the dermis and connects to the underlying muscle tissue. The hypodermis consists of major blood vessels and adipose cells. The information below describes the terminology used in referring to the integumentary system.

The epidermis and dermis make up the actual skin.
The epidermis and dermis are collectively called the **integument**.
The epidermis and dermis are also collectively called the **cutaneous layer**.
Therefore, the hypodermis is the **subcutaneous layer**.
When a patient is given an injection, the medicine needs to be placed near the
blood vessels, which is in the subcutaneous layer or hypodermis layer.
Hence the term subcutaneous injection or hence the term hypodermic needle.

The hypodermis is not considered to be a component of the integumentary system. However, it is always discussed when speaking of the integumentary system. The following table briefly describes the significance of the hypodermis.

	Hypodermis	Feature
1	**Hypodermis layer**	Consists of major blood vessels. Consists of adipocytes. This layer also contains the areolar cells that attach skin to the muscles.

CLEAVAGE LINES

The **cleavage lines** of the body are lines of tissue that correspond to the natural orientation of collagen fibers in the dermis. Many times, a surgeon, if possible, will make an incision that corresponds to the cleavage lines to reduce scarring.

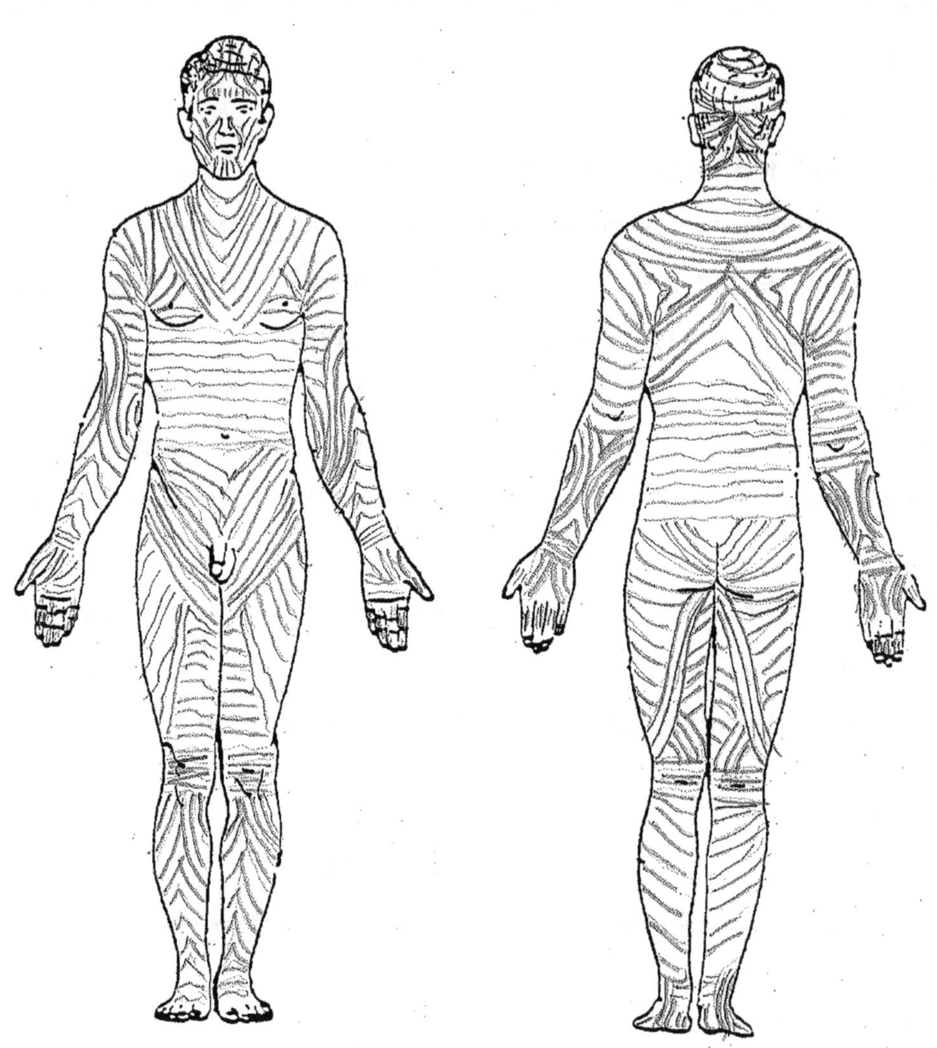

THE INTEGUMENTARY SYSTEM:
ADDITIONAL INFORMATION

Below is some additional information regarding the integumentary system. Your instructor may add to this list.

1. The integumentary system consists of more than just skin.

2. Fingerprints are found at the junction of the epidermis with the dermis.

3. The skin is an organ because it consists of cells and tissues that work together to perform a task.

4. Cells of the epidermis migrate from the stratum basale layer to the stratum corneum layer.

5. The dye associated with tattoos must be injected into the dermis; otherwise the tattoo will fade away as the cells of the epidermis migrate to the surface and are sloughed off.

6. Dandruff results when sheets of cells of the stratum corneum are sloughed off all at once.

7. Acne is due to excess activity of the sebaceous glands.

8. Melanocytes are cells found in the stratum germinativum area that produce **melanin**, which creates skin color and the "tan" look. Melanin protects the skin from harmful sun radiation.

9. Knowing the direction of cleavage lines within a specific area of the skin is important for surgical operations, particularly cosmetic surgery. If a surgeon has a choice about where and in what direction to place an incision, he or she may choose to cut in the direction of the cleavage lines. Incisions made parallel to the cleavage lines may heal better and produce less scarring than those that cut across.

10. The existing hair on your head does not turn gray. As you age, hair falls out. The new hair that comes in lacks pigment (which is an aging concept) and is typically finer than the hair you lost. This new hair gives the appearance of "hair turning gray."

11. The structures associated with the nail are:
     Lunula / Eponychium / Hyponychium / Lateral nail groove / Free edge

Chapter 4:   The Head and Neck Region

The following chapters are divided into major regions of the body. This chapter is the head and neck region. Each major chapter is further subdivided into topics labeled A, B, C, and D.   The major topics are as follows:

4 A. discusses the bones of that region

4 B. discusses the muscles of that region

4 C. discusses the blood vessels of that region

4 D. discusses the nerves of that region

4 E. discusses the viscera in the neck region.

4A.   The entire skeleton consists of 206 individual bones. Those 206 bones have numerous projections, prominences, depressions, holes, etc. Each protrusion or depression has a name (everything has a name!). Each part of a bone is not named just for exam purposes; each part has a specific name based on its structure or its function. This chapter concentrates on just the skull. Disease, malformation, or trauma to the head forms the bases for many specialties, such as: dentistry, maxillofacial surgery and rhinology to list a few.

4B.   The muscles of the face and scalp create the numerous facial expressions we exhibit. Most of these muscles are different than other skeletal muscles because most skeletal muscles originate and insert on a bone or bony structures. Most of the facial muscles insert in soft tissue such as fascia. The platysma and many facial muscles are fused together during embryonic times and therefore, during dissection, are very difficult to separate.

4C.   The major supply of blood to the head (specifically to the brain) is carried by the carotid arteries. The right common carotid artery branches from the brachiocephalic artery. The left common carotid artery arises directly from the aortic arch. In the area of the thyroid cartilage, the common carotid bifurcates to form the internal carotid and external carotid arteries. Both of these arteries will branch many times thus going to different parts of the skull and the brain. The external carotid artery branches to form the facial artery and the superficial temporal artery. The internal carotid artery supplies blood to the pituitary gland as well as the brain. In the base of the internal carotid artery are special cells that detect carbon dioxide concentrations and blood pressure. These special cells are called chemoreceptors and baroreceptors.

4D.   The chemical and biological processes (physiology) of the brain are very complex. However, the anatomy of the brain is actually fairly simple. Extremely detailed anatomy of the brain is discussed in a neuroanatomy class, of which this class is not.

4E.   The viscera of the neck region consists of endocrine organs (thyroid and parathyroid glands), respiratory organs (larynx and trachea), and organs associated with digestion (esophagus).

Chapter 4A: The Skull

The following table indicates the number of individual bones comprising just the skull and face.

Skull and Associated Bones	
Cranium	8
Face	14
Associated bones	6 auditory ossicles 1 hyoid
Total	**29**

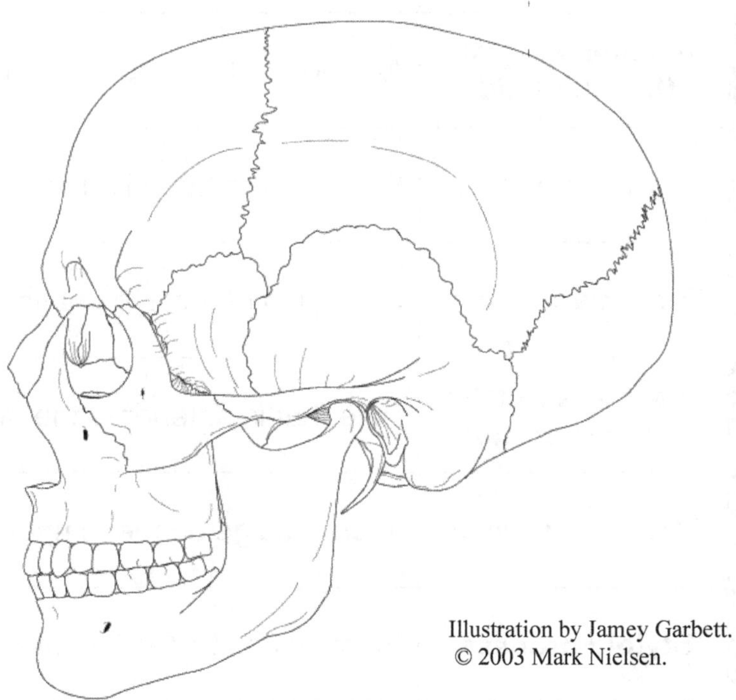

Illustration by Jamey Garbett.
© 2003 Mark Nielsen.

Lateral View

The following table lists the various bones and bone structures of the skull and face. While studying this table, examine pictures in your textbook.

	Bone or Bone Structure	Description
1	**Frontal bone**	Anterior to the parietal bone
2	**Parietal bone**	Posterior to the frontal bone
3	**Occipital bone**	Posterior to the parietal bones
4	**Temporal bone**	Inferior to the parietal bone
5	**Greater wing of the sphenoid**	Anterior to the temporal bone
6	**Zygomatic**	Bulge on the lateral edge of the face.
7	**Zygomatic arch**	Extension of the zygomatic
8	**External acoustic canal (meatus)**	Hole that is anterior to the mastoid process
9	**Mastoid process**	Inferior bulge on the temporal bone.
10	**Styloid process**	Pointy extension in the inferior aspect of the skull

ANTERIOR VIEW

The two following tables list the various bones and bone structures of the skull and face. While studying these tables, examine pictures in your textbook.

Bone or Bone Structure		Description
1	**Frontal bone**	Anterior bone of the cranium.
2	**Nasal bone**	Two bones that make up the bridge of the nose
3	**Maxilla bone**	Two bones that make up the upper jaw
4	**Anterior Nasal Spine**	Pointy projection at the anterior edge of the nasal septum
5	**Mandible bone**	Lower jaw
6	**Zygomatic**	Lateral bulges of the face but can be seen easily from the anterior view.

INFERIOR VIEW

Bone or Bone Structure		Description
1	**Foramen magnum**	Huge hole in the occipital bone
2	**Basioccipital**	Bridge of bone anterior to the foramen magnum
3	**Occipital condyles**	Bulges that are lateral to the foramen magnum
4	**Posterior palatine bone**	Posterior bone of the palate
5	**Anterior palatine**	Anterior to the posterior palatine. Not a separate bone. This is part of the maxilla.

NASAL CAVITY AND EYE SOCKET

The tables below list the various bones and bone structures of the nasal cavity and the eye socket. While studying these tables, examine pictures in your textbook.

NASAL CAVITY

	Bone or Bone Structure	Description
1	Vomer	Inferior bone of the nasal septum
2	Perpendicular Plate of the Ethmoid	Superior bone of the nasal septum
3	Nasal Conchae	Bulges lateral to the nasal septum. The nasal conchae are identified in the "Additional Information" section.

EYE SOCKET

	Bone or Bone Structure	Description
1	Sphenoid bone	Makes up the posterior wall
2	Frontal bone	Makes up the roof of eye socket
3	Zygomatic	Makes up the lateral wall
4	Maxilla bone	Makes up a portion of the floor
5	Lacrimal bone	Makes up medial wall (anterior to ethmoid)
6	Ethmoid bone	Makes up medial wall (posterior to lacrimal)
7	Palatine bone	Deep in the orbit, between the ethmoid, the maxilla, and the sphenoid (not easily seen).

INTERNAL VIEW

The following table lists the various bones and bone structures of the internal skull. While studying this table, examine pictures in your textbook.

	Bone or Bone Structure	Description
1	**Foramen magnum**	Huge hole in the occipital bone
2	**Clivus**	Anterior to the foramen magnum. Forms a natural "slide" from the dorsum sella towards the foramen magnum.
3	**Dorsum sella**	Posterior ridge of the sella turcica
4	**Hypophyseal fossa**	Deep depression anterior to the dorsum sella
5	**Tuberculum sellae**	Ridge that is anterior to the hypophyseal fossa
6	**Crista galli**	Pointy projection in of the ethmoid bone in the anterior cranial fossa.
7	**Cribriform plate**	Plate that surrounds the crista galli. This is a horizontal plate of the ethmoid.
8	**Petrous portion of the temporal bone**	Large ridge lateral to the foramen magnum. It runs at an oblique angle laterally from the clivus.

The following table lists the various foramen of the anterior view. While studying this table, examine pictures in your textbook.

	Foramen / Fissure / Notch	Description
1	Supraorbital notch	A notch on the superior orbit of the eye socket. This may be a foramen in some skulls.
2	Infraorbital foramen	Huge holes inferior to the eye socket on the maxilla
3	Mental foramen	Holes in the body of the mandible
4	Superior orbital fissure	Superior slit in the eye socket
5	Inferior orbital fissure	Inferior slit in the eye socket
6	Optic foramen (canal)	Round hole located at the back of the eye socket
7	Lacrimal foramen	Hole located at the distal end of the lacrimal bone

The following table lists the various foramen of the inferior view. While studying this table, examine pictures in your textbook.

Foramen / Fissure / Notch		Description
1	Foramen magnum	The largest foramen of the skull
2	Foramen lacerum	The foramen lateral to the basioccipital
3	Foramen ovale	The foramen lateral to the foramen lacerum
4	Foramen spinosum	The small foramen slightly posterior to the foramen ovale
5	Carotid foramen (canal)	The foramen posterior to the foramen spinosum
6	Jugular foramen	The foramen posterior to the carotid foramen
7	Condyloid foramen	The foramen posterior to the occipital condyles
8	Hypoglossal foramen (canal)	The foramen passing superior to the occipital condyles. Also can be seen on the lateral wall of the foramen magnum.
9	Anterior palatine foramen (incisive foramen)	The foramen located posterior to the incisor teeth on the anterior palatine.
10	Greater palatine foramen	The foramen located at the lateral edges of the posterior palatine bone.
11	Stylomastoid foramen	Located immediately posterior to the styloid process.

FORAMEN AND FISSURES (INTERNAL VIEW)

The following table lists the various foramen of the internal view. While studying this table, examine pictures in your textbook.

	Foramen / Fissure / Notch	Description
1	**Foramen magnum**	Large hole in the occipital bone
2	**Foramen lacerum**	This foramen is lateral to the dorsum sella
3	**Foramen ovale**	This foramen is lateral to the foramen lacerum
4	**Foramen spinosum**	This foramen is posterior to the foramen ovale
5	**Carotid foramen (canal)**	Go posterior to the foramen spinosum you will find a channel that goes toward and joins the foramen lacerum. This is why the carotid foramen is sometimes called the carotid canal.
6	**Jugular foramen**	This foramen is posterior to the carotid foramen. It is posterior to the petrous portion of the temporal bone. This foramen is the large hole on the posterior edge of the petrous portion of the temporal bone.
7	**Internal acoustic canal (meatus)**	This canal is superior to the jugular foramen. This canal is still on the posterior side of the petrous portion of the temporal bone.
8	**Foramen rotundum**	This foramen is anterior to the foramen ovale.
9	**Olfactory foramina**	These foramina are on the cribriform plate (cribriform plate foramina)
10	**Optic foramen**	These are located on the lateral edges of the tuberculum sellae.

SUTURES

The following table lists the various sutures of the skull. While studying this table, examine pictures in your textbook.

	Sutures	Description
1	**Sagittal**	Connects the two parietal bones together.
2	**Coronal**	Connects the frontal bone with the parietal bones.
3	**Lambdoidal**	Connects the parietal bones with the occipital bone.
4	**Squamosal**	Connects the temporal bone with the parietal bones.
5	**Sphenosquamosal**	Connects the greater wing of the sphenoid with the temporal bone.

Formerly, the temporal bone was called the squamosal bone.

Squamous means flat and the squamosal bone is a relatively flat bone of the skull when compared to the curved frontal, parietal, and occipital bones.

Therefore, the suture associated was called the squamosal suture.

As the years went by, the squamosal bone name was changed to temporal bone.

However, the name of the suture remained.

Mandible

The following table lists the various structures of the mandible. While studying this table, examine pictures in your textbook.

Mandibular Structures		Description
1	**Mandibular condyle (condylar process)**	The rounded, posterior process of the mandible that forms the hinge of the jaw joint.
2	**Mandibular fossa**	The depression in the temporal bone that forms the socket for the hinge joint of the mandible. This is not a part of the mandible but is part of the mandibular hinge.
3	**Mandibular notch**	Curved area anterior to the mandibular condyle.
4	**Coronoid process**	A pointy projection anterior to the mandibular notch
5	**Ramus**	This area of the mandible extends from the mandibular notch to the inferior border of the mandible.
6	**Angle of the mandible**	This is the posterior edge of the mandible in the area of the junction of the ramus and the body of the mandible.
7	**Body**	This is the main portion of the mandible extending from the left ramus to the right ramus.
8	**Mental protuberance**	Located in the area of the dimple of the chin. If you move your finger side to side and you can feel this bump.
9	**Alveolar processes**	These are tooth sockets. They feel like bumps on the mandible and maxilla.

TEETH

We study the teeth at this time only because they are attached to the mandible and the maxilla. We will study the teeth in more detail when we get to the digestive chapter.

The average adult will have 28-32 teeth. If the adult has all four of their "wisdom teeth", they will have 32 teeth. If they are missing their "wisdom teeth" they will only have 28 teeth.

The "wisdom teeth" are the most posterior molars of the mandible and maxilla.

Be sure to examine figures in your textbook while studying the table below.

	Teeth	Description
1	**Incisors**	The four front teeth (4 per jaw).
2	**Cuspids**	Lateral to the lateral incisors (2 per jaw).
3	**Bicuspids**	Lateral to the cuspids (4 per jaw). Also called the premolars.
4	**Molars**	Posterior to the bicuspids (6 per jaw) The last molar has been dubbed as the "wisdom tooth."

Many times, dentists use the term **distal** rather than lateral or posterior when referring to the positioning of the teeth. For example, the cuspids are distal to the lateral incisors. The bicuspids are distal to the cuspids. The molars are distal to the bicuspids.

The Fetal Skull

Fetal Skull		Description
1	**Anterior fontanel**	The fibrous membrane in the area between the frontal bone and the parietal bones.
2	**Posterior fontanel**	The fibrous membrane in the area between the occipital bone and the parietal bones.

The anterior fontanel is also called the frontal fontanel and is known as the "baby's soft spot" in layman's terms.

In the fetus, the sutures have not completely formed yet.

This allows for compression of the skull as it is passing through the birth canal.

At the time of birth, the only thing that is protecting the baby's brain in that area is the fibrous membrane (dura mater).

As the child ages, the bones grow closer together to ultimately form a strong suture.

The anterior fontanel closes in 90% of the children within 19 months.

THE SKULL:
ADDITIONAL INFORMATION

Here is some additional information regarding the skull bones. Your instructor may add to this list.

1. Foramen means hole. Foramina is plural.

2. Fossa means depression.

3. Condyle means rounded process that articulates with another bone.

4. The petrous portion of the temporal bone angles medial to lateral going toward the posterior portion of the skull.

5. The pituitary gland sits in the hypophyseal fossa of the sella turcica. Sella turcica is Latin that means, "Turkish saddle."

6. The sella turcica consists of the three parts (that we study) and is a part of the sphenoid bone.

7. Fontanel is Latin for "little fountain." This is because you can put your finger on an infant's skull in the area of the anterior fontanel and you can feel the blood pulse (flow like a fountain).

8. A sunken fontanel could mean the infant is dehydrated and a bulging fontanel could mean there is an increase in intracranial pressure.

9. Zygomatic is Latin for "like a yoke." This is in reference to the yoke that holds to oxen together. The yoke of the skull is made of the left zygomatic, the maxillary bone, and the right zygomatic.

10. Lambdoid suture is in reference to the Greek letter lambda used in mathematics. The lambdoid (lambdoidal) suture forms an upside down curve that merges with the sagittal suture. This is the lambda symbol:

λ

This is a portion of the sagittal suture

This is the left portion of the suture

This is the right portion of the suture

11. There is only 1 frontal bone.

12. The frontal bone, parietal bones, and the occipital bone make up the **calvaria** (skull cap).

13. There are 2 parietal bones.

14. There is 1 occipital bone.

15. There are 2 temporal bones.

16. There is only 1 sphenoid bone. It extends from the left greater wing to the right greater wing.

17. There are 2 zygomatic bones. They provide connection between the maxilla and the temporal bones. Zygo is Latin that means, "like a yoke."

18. The zygomatic arch is made of the zygomatic process of the temporal bone and the temporal process of the zygomatic bone.

19. The external acoustic canal is also called: external auditory canal / external auditory meatus / external acoustic meatus.

20. The mastoid process is not a separate bone. It is a part of the temporal bone. Huge neck muscles attach to it.

21. The styloid process serves as an attachment point for muscles of the tongue, larynx, and the hyoid bone.

22. There are 2 nasal bones making up the "bridge" of the nose.

23. There are 2 maxilla bones. There is a suture in the philtrum area. This is called the intermaxillary suture.

24. The anterior nasal spine is a part of the maxilla bone.

25. There is 1 mandible bone.

26. In layman's terms, the zygomatic is the cheek bone.

27. There is 1 vomer.

28. The perpendicular plate of the ethmoid is a part of the ethmoid bone. It is perpendicular to the ethmoid and extends into the cranial cavity forming the crista galli.

29. The lacrimal bone has the lacrimal foramen at its distal end.

30. The ethmoid bone consists of the perpendicular plate of the ethmoid, cribriform plate, and crista galli.

31. The spinal cord passes through the foramen magnum to go to and from the brain.

32. The basioccipital makes up the base of the occipital bone.

33. Vertebra number one (atlas) articulates with the occipital condyles.

34. The posterior palatine is a separate bone and is sometimes simply called the palatine bone.

35. The anterior palatine is not a separate bone. It is a part of the maxilla and is sometimes called the palatine process of the maxilla.

36. The clivus forms a slant extending from the foramen magnum area to the dorsum sella.

37. The dorsum sella, hypophyseal fossa, and tuberculum sellae collectively make up the sella turcica. The pituitary gland (hypophysis) sits in the hypophyseal fossa.

38. The crista galli is an extension of the perpendicular plate of the ethmoid. It serves as the anterior attachment for a portion of the brain.

39. The cribriform plate consists of numerous foramen (olfactory foramina) through which the olfactory nerves passes.

40. Housed inside the petrous portion of the temporal bone are the cochlea and vestibular apparatus of the ear.

41. The supraorbital notch is sometimes called the supraorbital foramen.

42. The infraorbital artery and nerve pass through infraorbital foramen.

43. The mental artery and nerve pass through the mental foramen.

44. Cranial nerves pass through superior orbital fissure (discussed later).

45. The optic foramen is also called the optic canal. The optic nerves pass through this foramen.

46. Tears drain through the lacrimal foramen into the nasal cavity.

47. The foramen lacerum has jagged edges, hence the term lacerum (lacerate).

48. The foramen ovale is usually oval shaped.

49. The carotid foramen is also called the carotid canal. In the internal view, the canal joins with the foramen lacerum.

50. Passing through the jugular foramen is the jugular vein that transports blood from the brain area back to the heart.

51. Nerves that control the tongue pass through the hypoglossal foramen.

52. The anterior palatine foramen is also called the incisive foramen because of its proximity to the incisor teeth.

53. There are also smaller foramen in close proximity to the greater palatine foramen called the lesser palatine foramen.

54. The vestibulocochlear nerve leaves the cochlea within the petrous portion of the temporal bone via the internal acoustic canal and goes to the brain for the interpretation of hearing.

55. The mandibular condyle is sometimes called the condylar process or the head of the mandible.

56. The TMJ
    a. The mandibular condyle is a part of the mandible.
    b. The mandibular fossa is a part of the temporal bone.
    c. The combination of these results in the temporal-mandibular joint (TMJ)

57. When the mandible is closed, the coronoid process is obscured by the zygomatic arch.

58. There are 3 pairs of nasal conchae. 1. Superior nasal conchae
                                          2. Middle nasal conchae
                                          3. Inferior nasal conchae

Chapter 4B: The Skull and Face Muscles

Use your textbook to examine figures of select muscles of the face and neck.

Muscle	Description
	Muscles of the Face
1 **Frontalis**	This muscle covers the frons area.
2 **Orbicularis oculi**	This muscle encircles the orbit of the eye.
3 **Nasalis**	These muscles cover the "bridge" of the nose.
4 **Orbicularis oris**	This muscle encircles the mouth.
5 **Mentalis**	This muscle is in the center of the anterior chin.
6 **Depressor labii inferioris**	This muscle is lateral to the mentalis.
7 **Depressor anguli oris**	This muscle is lateral to the depressor labii inferioris.

Use your textbook to examine figures of the muscles of the face and neck.

	Muscle	Description
		Muscles of the Face
8	**Zygomaticus minor**	This muscle extends from the orbicularis oris to the zygomatic bone. It is superior to the zygomaticus major. It is smaller in width than the zygomaticus major.
9	**Zygomaticus major**	This muscle extends from the corner of the mouth to the zygomatic bone. It is inferior to the zygomaticus minor.
10	**Risorius**	This muscle extends from the corner of the mouth to straight posterior toward the ramus of the mandible. It is inferior to the zygomaticus major.
11	**Masseter**	This muscle is superficial to the ramus of the mandible.
12	**Levator labii superioris alaeque nasi**	This muscle extends from the orbicularis oris, passes near the ala of the nose and inserts close the medial corner of the eye socket. Sometimes a portion extends directly from the ala of the nose to the medial corner of the eye.
13	**Levator labii superioris**	This muscle is lateral to the levator labii superioris alaeque nasi.
14	**Buccinator**	This muscle is deep and slightly anterior to the masseter.
15	**Occipitalis**	This is a posterior muscle located on the occipital bone.
16	**Temporalis**	This is a lateral muscle located on the temporal bone.

THE NECK MUSCLES

Use your textbook to examine figures of the muscles of the face and neck.

Muscle	Description
Muscles of the Neck	
1 **Platysma**	This thin, sheet-like muscle covers the entire anterior neck. It extends from the clavicle to the mandible.
2 **Sternocleidomastoid**	This is a huge muscle that extends from the clavicle and the sternum and merges to insert on the mastoid process.
3 **Trapezius**	This is mainly an upper back muscle but it also extends through the posterior neck to the occipital region.

Identify the muscles in the posterior neck that are located between the trapezius and the sternocleidomastoid.

Muscle	Description
4 **Anterior scalene**	
5 **Middle scalene**	Begin at the inferior end of the clavicular head of the sternocleidomastoid and identify the scalenes by moving superior and posterior.
6 **Posterior scalene**	
7 **Levator scapulae**	Superior to the posterior scalene.
8 **Splenius capitis**	Superior to the levator scapulae

Use your textbook to examine figures of the muscles of the face and neck.

	Muscle	Description
		Muscles of the Neck
9	**Sternohyoid**	This is an anterior neck muscle
10	**Omohyoid**	This muscle is deep to the sternohyoid. It extends from the hyoid bone and runs oblique to the clavicle.
11	**Digastric**	This muscle extends from the hyoid bone to the area at the center of the mandible.
12	**Mylohyoid**	This muscle is deep to the digastric and forms the floor of the mouth.

Below is some additional information regarding the muscles of the head and neck region. Your instructor may add to this list.

1. The sternocleidomastoid muscle has 3 points of attachment:
    a. Mastoid process of the skull
    b. Clavicle – "cleido"
    c. Sterno – manubrium of the sternum

2. Levator labii superioris alaeque nasi:
    a. Levator means to elevate.
    b. Labii means lips
    c. Superioris means a superior muscle (in location)
    d. Alaeque is in reference to the ala of the nose
    e. Nasi is in reference to the nose area

3. The occipitalis and frontalis are connected across the surface of the scalp via dense tissue called epicranial aponeurosis.

4. Some anatomists consider the occipitalis and the frontalis to be one muscle (the occipitofrontalis), with two bellies (the occipitalis belly and the frontalis belly).

5. The trapezius muscle is an upper back muscle that extends from the occipital and thoracic vertebrae and inserts on the clavicle and the scapula. This muscle extends over the shoulder and can be partially seen from an anterior view.

Chapter 4C: The Blood Vessels

Examine figures in your textbook while studying the following tables.

	Blood vessel	Description
1	**Common carotid artery**	The right common carotid artery branches off the brachiocephalic artery. The left common carotid artery branches off the aortic arch.
2	**External carotid a**	Branches off the common carotid at the level of the thyroid cartilage and goes to the superficial regions of the skull.
3	**Facial a**	Branches off the external carotid a at the level of the mandible. It goes across the edge of the mandible a few centimeters anterior to the angle of the mandible.
4	**Superficial temporal a**	Extends from the external carotid a to the mid portion of the temporal bone and then branches to other parts of the skull.
5	**Occipital a**	Branches off the external carotid a at the same level as the facial a. It supplies blood to the occipital region.

	Blood vessel	Description
6	Internal carotid artery	Branches off the common carotid at the level of the thyroid cartilage and goes deep into the skull through the carotid canal. Branches to form the middle cerebral a and vessels that surround the pituitary gland (cerebral arterial circle).
7	Middle cerebral a	Branches numerous times to supply blood to various aspects of the brain.
8	Cerebral arterial circle	Consists of numerous blood vessels surrounding the pituitary gland.
9	Vertebral a	First branch off the subclavian arteries (a few centimeters lateral to the base of the common carotid arteries) and pass through the transverse foramen of the cervical vertebrae to deliver blood to the cerebral arterial circle of the pituitary gland.
10	Basilar a	The left and right vertebral arteries merge to form the basilar a. The basilar a also supplies the vessels of the cerebral arterial circle.

Below is some additional information regarding the blood vessels of the head and neck region. Your instructor may add to this list.

1. The cerebral arterial circle is known as the circle of Willis in layman's terms.

2. If there is blockage in the right carotid artery, blood will still deliver nutrients to the pituitary gland via the left internal carotid artery and the left and right vertebral arteries.

3. If there is blockage in the right vertebral artery, blood will still deliver nutrients to the pituitary gland via the left and right internal carotid arteries and the left vertebral artery.

4. The blood vessels associated with the cerebral arterial circle are more numerous than the ones listed in the previous table.

Chapter 4D: The Brain

The highlighted part of the chart will be discussed in this chapter and the parts that are not highlighted will be discussed in later chapters.

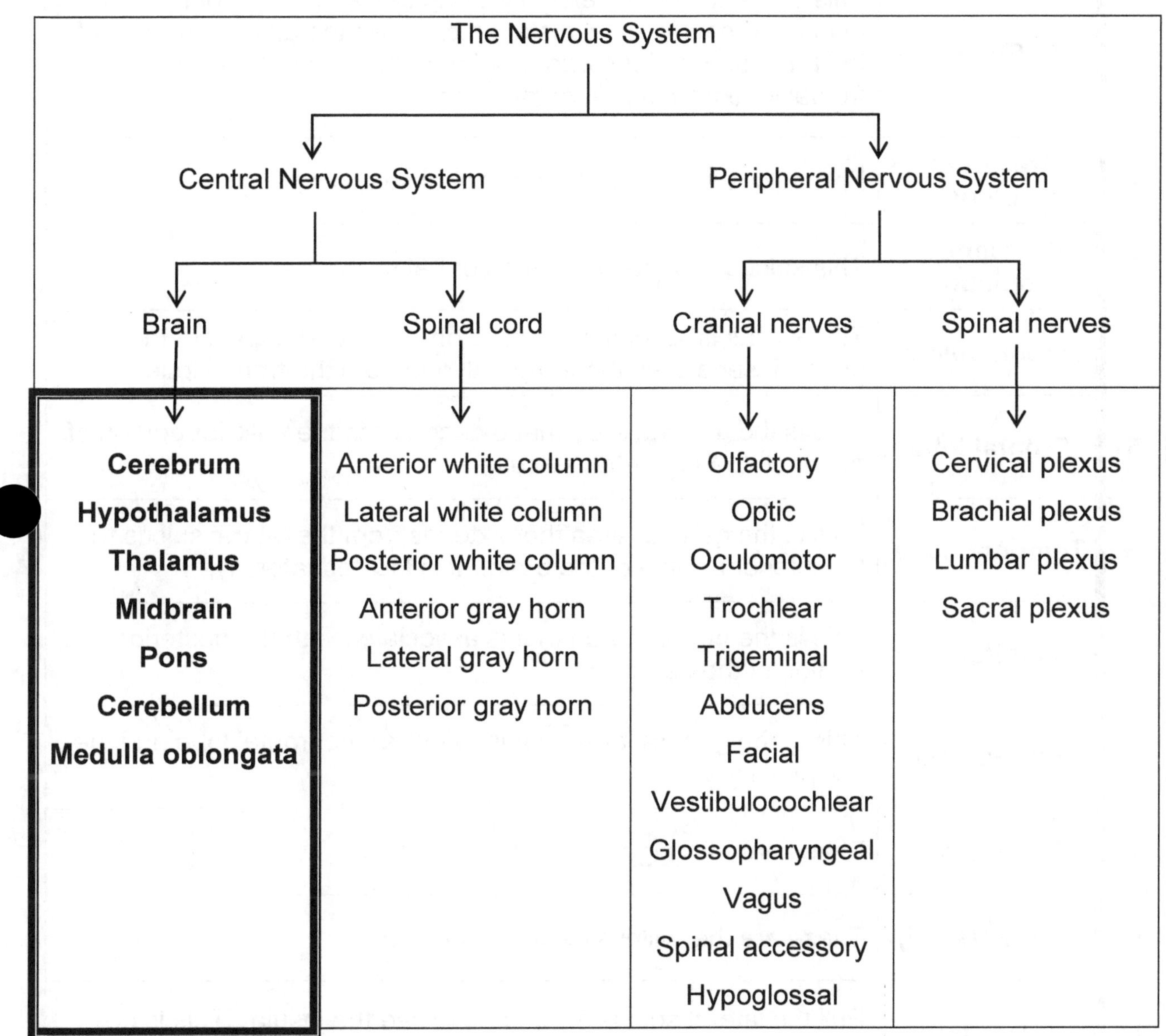

Study pictures of the brain while examining the table below.

	External brain	Description
1	Central sulcus	This sulcus extends vertically along the lateral side of the brain at approximately equal distance between the anterior portion of the brain and the posterior portion of the brain. It separates the frontal lobe from the parietal lobes.
2	Precentral sulcus	This sulcus is anterior to the central sulcus.
3	Postcentral sulcus	This sulcus is posterior to the central sulcus.
4	Lateral sulcus	This sulcus is an oblique sulcus on the lateral aspect of the brain. It separates the temporal lobe from the frontal lobe.
5	Frontal lobe	This is the general area that extends from the anterior portion of the brain to the central sulcus.
6	Temporal lobe	This is the general area that extends from the lateral sulcus to the inferior portion of the brain. It is located laterally.
7	Occipital lobe	This is the general area that is associated with the posterior portion of the cerebrum.
8	Parietal lobe	This is the general area that is between the frontal lobe and the occipital lobe.
9	Gyrus (gyri)	These are the ridges of the brain.
10	Sulcus (sulci)	These are the valleys between the gyri.
11	Insula	Pull the lateral sulcus apart a bit to see the insula. This is deep to the lateral sulcus.

EXTERNAL BRAIN ---- SELECT FUNCTIONS

The following table identifies a few select functions of the previous brain structures. This is not a complete list of functions.

	External brain	Function
1	**Frontal lobe**	Voluntary motor actions / concentration / verbal communication / decision making / personality
2	**Temporal lobe**	Hearing / smell
3	**Occipital lobe**	Vision / visual memories
4	**Parietal lobe**	Interpretation of touch / pressure / pain / temperature
5	**Insula**	Perhaps involved with taste and memory

Study pictures of the brain while examining the table below.

	Sagittal Brain	Description
1	**Longitudinal fissure**	This is the real deep sulcus between the hemispheres of the brain, which runs along the midline.
2	**Corpus callosum**	This is a bundle of fiber tracts that connects the left hemisphere with the right hemisphere. It consists of a posterior portion called the **splenium**. Anterior to the splenium is the **body**. Anterior to the area of the body is the **genu**. Curving from the genu posteriorly again is the **rostrum.**
3	**Limbic system**	This is a system of nerves located in the cingulate gyrus
4	**Cingulate gyrus**	This is a gyrus superior to the corpus callosum and basically outlining the corpus callosum.
5	**Parahippocampal gyrus**	This is an extension of the cingulate gyrus that curves around the splenium of the corpus callosum and enters into the temporal lobe.
6	**Hippocampus**	This is a bundle of nerves that lies on the superior edge of the parahippocampal gyrus and extends around the superior surface of the fornix, curving posteriorly at the anterior end of the fornix terminating at the mammillary body.
7	**Fornix**	This is a bundle of nerves that lies along the inferior edge of the corpus callosum and curves almost to the rostrum of the corpus callosum.

Study pictures of the brain while examining the table below.

Sagittal Brain		Description
8	**Lateral ventricles**	This is a ventricle that is located between the fornix area and the corpus callosum. There is one located in each hemisphere.
9	**Septum pellucidum**	This is membranous material that divides the left lateral ventricle with the right lateral ventricle. The ventricles are also called ventricle 1 and ventricle 2.
10	**Thalamus**	A relatively circular area inferior to the fornix region.
11	**Choroid plexus**	This is a network of blood vessels located at the inferior edge of the fornix and also the superior edge. It is also located in the 4th ventricle area.
12	**Hypothalamus**	This is an area that slants anteriorly from the inferior edge of the thalamus.
13	**Pituitary gland**	This gland is connected to the hypothalamus via the **infundibulum**. This is a stalk-like structure that connects the pituitary to the hypothalamus. The function of the infundibulum is more than simply an attachment structure. The function is discussed in detail in a physiology course.
14	**Pons**	This is a rather large bulge of nerve tissue inferior to the midbrain.
15	**Midbrain**	This is the nerve tissue that is between the pons and the thalamus.

Study pictures of the brain while examining the table below.

	Sagittal Brain	Description
16	Medulla oblongata	This is a subtle bulge of nerve tissue inferior to the pons.
17	4th ventricle	This is a cavity located between the pons area and the cerebellum.
18	3rd ventricle	This is the cavity located within the thalamus.
19	Corpora quadrigemina	This is the posterior portion (posterior edge) of the midbrain. It consists of two bulges: Superior colliculus Inferior colliculus
20	Pineal gland	This is a small gland located superior to the superior colliculus and inferior to the splenium of the corpus callosum.
21	Interthalmic adhesion	This is a small mass of tissue in the center of the thalamus that connects the right thalamus with the left thalamus. It passes through the 3rd ventricle.
22	Mammillary body	This is a small mass of tissue located on the posterior edge of the hypothalamus.
23	Cerebellum	Located posterior to the pons area and inferior to the occipital lobe.
24	Spinal cord	This extends from the medulla oblongata to the coccygeal region.

The following table identifies a few select functions of the previous brain structures. This is not a complete list of functions.

	Sagittal Brain	Function
1	Corpus callosum	A bundle of nerves that connect the right and left hemispheres
2	Limbic system	The system of nerves that are involved in long-term memory.
3	Cingulate gyrus	All are part of the limbic system and are involved with long-term memory.
4	Parahippocampal gyrus	
5	Hippocampus	
9	Septum pellucidum	Membranous material that forms a wall between the left lateral ventricle and the right lateral ventricle.
10	Thalamus	All sensory information arrives and is stored in the thalamus (except for olfaction). Consists of a portion of the RAS.
11	Choroid plexus	Cells that produce CSF (cerebrospinal fluid), which bathes the central nervous system thus providing some protection.
12	Hypothalamus	Controls the autonomic nerves / controls the endocrine system / regulates body temperature / controls emotions / controls some behaviors / regulates thirst / involved in the circadian rhythm.
13	Pituitary gland	Produces and releases numerous hormones.
14	Pons	Regulates the rate and depth of breathing.

The following table continues the identification of a few select functions of the previous brain structures. This is not a complete list of functions.

	Sagittal Brain	Function
15	**Midbrain**	Contains a portion of the RAS / maintains involuntary muscle tone
16	**Medulla oblongata**	Regulates rhythmic breathing and heart rate / regulates blood pressure by changing the diameter of blood vessels / involuntary sneezing, coughing, and vomiting.
17	**Corpora quadrigemina**	Superior colliculus: Allows us to turn our head in the direction of a visual stimulus. Inferior colliculus: Allows us to turn our head in the direction of an auditory stimulus.
18	**Pineal gland**	Secretes melatonin, which regulates the circadian rhythms (day-night cycles)
19	**Interthalmic adhesion**	Connects the right thalamus with the left thalamus.
20	**Mammillary body**	Involved in the feeding reflexes of licking, swallowing, and chewing.
21	**Cerebellum**	Coordinates and "fine tunes" skeletal muscle activity / stores memory of some movements
22	**Spinal cord**	Transmits information to and from the cerebrum / consists of 31 pairs of spinal nerves, which transmits information to and from the spinal cord.
23	**RAS**	Reticular activating system: This is the system of nerves that keep us alert (conscious).

DIVISIONS

        Anatomists have further subdivided the brain for understanding purposes. There are 5 major embryonic divisions of the brain that will form some of the structures identified in previous tables referring to the sagittal view of the brain.

	Brain Division	Associated Structures
1	Telencephalon	Cerebrum
2	Diencephalon	Hypothalamus / Thalamus / Pineal gland
3	Mesencephalon	Midbrain
4	Metencephalon	Pons / Cerebellum
5	Myelencephalon	Medulla Oblongata

THE CEREBRAL NUCLEI

There is a special group of nerves deep in the brain that are collectively called the cerebral nuclei. These are located between the base of the brain and the lateral ventricle. They are seen using a frontal cut of the brain. The following table describes the location of the various components of the cerebral nuclei.

	Cerebral Nuclei Structure	Description
1	Caudate nucleus	Small mass of nerves located lateral to the lateral ventricle.
2	Putamen	A larger mass of nerves located inferior and lateral to the caudate nucleus.
3	Globus pallidus	A similar size of a mass of nerves as the putamen and located along the medial edge of the putamen.
4	Amygdaloid body	A small mass of nerves located inferior to the putamen. This is located at the terminal end of the hippocampus.
5	Substantia nigra	A small of nerves located at the superior edge of the pons. (not a part of the cerebral nuclei but can be seen in a frontal view with the components of the cerebral nuclei)

THE CEREBRAL NUCLEI --- SELECT FUNCTIONS

The following table identifies a few select functions of the components of the cerebral nuclei.

	Cerebral nuclei structure	Function
1	Caudate nucleus	Releases acetylcholine for muscle contraction.
2	Putamen	Releases GABA (gamma amino butyric acid). Regulates the level of dopamine release from the substantia nigra.
3	Globus pallidus	Controls muscle tone of the appendicular muscles.
4	Amygdaloid body	Associated with long-term memory and emotional balance.
5	Substantia nigra	Releases dopamine, which regulates the level of acetylcholine release from the caudate nucleus.

The following table describes detailed functions of the cerebral nuclei in relation to specific nerve disorders.

Nerve Disorder		Action
1	Normal action	The cerebral cortex initiates the impulse to get a muscle to contract. An impulse is sent to the substantial nigra and the caudate nucleus. The caudate nucleus releases acetylcholine in order for a muscle to contract. The substantia nigra releases dopamine, which controls the amount of acetylcholine released from the caudate nucleus.
Parkinson's disease:		
Patients with Parkinson's disease show a decrease in substantia nigra activity. Therefore, there is very little dopamine released. Therefore, without adequate dopamine, the release of acetylcholine from the caudate nucleus is out of control. Since the acetylcholine is out of control, muscle contraction will be out of control, hence the "shakes" of voluntary muscles.		
2	Normal action	The putamen releases GABA. This chemical controls the release of dopamine. With dopamine under control, the ultimate release of acetylcholine from the caudate nucleus will be under control. The patient will have normal muscle contraction.
Huntington's disease:		
Patients with Huntington's disease show a decrease in putamen activity. Therefore, the level of GABA is decreased. This results in a lack of control over dopamine. A lack of control over dopamine results in excess dopamine activity. Excess dopamine activity results in too much control over acetylcholine release. This in effect, decreases acetylcholine function. Therefore, muscle contraction is diminished.		

The following table describes detailed functions of the cerebral nuclei in relation to specific nerve disorders.

Nerve Disorder		Action
3	**Normal action**	The globus pallidus functions to adjust muscle tone, specifically with the appendicular muscles.

Carbon monoxide poisoning:

Carbon monoxide has been found to cause damage to the globus pallidus. Therefore, the afflicted patient loses all muscle tone. Carbon monoxide also deprives the tissues of the body of oxygen, hence death.

| 4 | **Normal action** | Long-term memory is stored in the limbic system of which the amygdaloid body is a part of (located at the terminal end of the hippocampus). The release of acetylcholine from the hippocampus area seems to be involved in long-term memory. |

<u>Alzheimer's disease</u>

 Patients with Alzheimer's disease lack the enzymes necessary for the release of acetylcholine from the limbic system. Therefore, without acetylcholine from the limbic system, memory loss occurs. It also appears that the protein molecules of the amygdaloid body (amyloid protein) become all twisted and tangled in patients with Alzheimer's. This is known as a neurofibrillary tangle. Due to this, the nerves in the amygdaloid region begin to degenerate.

THE MENINGES

The following table describes the features of the central nervous system that are involved in providing protection for the brain and the spinal cord.

	Meninges	Description
1	**Meninges**	The meninges are three layers of membranous material that surround the brain and spinal cord.
2	**Pia mater**	This layer immediately covers the surface of the brain and spinal cord.
3	**Arachnoid mater**	This layer is superficial to the pia mater. There is a space between the pia mater and the arachnoid mater called the **subarachnoid space.** Cerebral spinal fluid (CSF) flows in this area.
		Cerebrospinal fluid (produced by the choroid plexus) flows between the pia mater and the arachnoid mater.
4	**Dura mater**	This layer is superficial to the arachnoid mater. It is the most superficial layer of the meninges. It is adjacent to the inside lining of the skull and spinal cord. There is a space between the arachnoid mater and the dura mater called the **subdural space**.
		Protecting the brain and spinal cord are these structures: Meninges / CSF / Skull and Vertebral bones

The following table continues the description of the meningeal layers. Be sure to find pictures in your textbook that shows the structures being described.

Meninges		Description
5	**Meningeal layer**	The dura mater consists of these two layers. The meningeal layer splits off the dura mater in the area of the longitudinal fissure and enters into the longitudinal fissure thus forming the **falx cerebri**.
	Endosteal layer	The endosteal layer splits off the dura mater in the area of the longitudinal fissure and continues lining the inside lining of the skull.
Venous blood flows from the brain and merges in the area of the longitudinal fissure forming the superior sagittal sinus.		
6	**Tentorium cerebelli**	This is an extension of the falx cerebri. It branches transversally and covers the base of the brain and part of it covers the superior portion of the cerebellum.

Below is some additional information regarding the brain. Your instructor may add to this list.

1. The brain and spinal cord comprise the central nervous system.

2. You can feel the dura mater of the meninges in the anterior fontanel region of an infant's skull.

3. The hypothalamus regulates:
    a. Body temperature
    b. Thirst drives
    c. Behavioral drives
    d. Releases some hormones

4. The midbrain is located between the pons and the thalamus.

5. The brainstem consists of:
    a. Midbrain
    b. Pons
    c. Medulla oblongata

6. The fornix is a bundle of nerves that curve under the corpus callosum and extend to the mammillary bodies located on the posterior edge of the hypothalamus.

7. A portion of the limbic system is located in a gyrus that is superior to the corpus callosum.

8. Corpus callosum is Latin that means, "body / hard."

9. Hippocampus is Latin that means, "seahorse."

10. Amygdaloid is Greek that means "almond shape."

Chapter 4E: The Viscera

The following table describes the cervical viscera. The cervical viscera can be subdivided into 3 main areas:

1.   Endocrine
2.   Respiratory
3.   Alimentary

Cervical Viscera	
Thyroid gland	Located about cervical 5 through thoracic 1. Consists of 2 major lobes connected via the isthmus. Lies on the trachea. Produces hormones (discussed in physiology).
Parathyroid glands	Four small glands located on the posterior side of the thyroid gland. Two are located on the superior portion of the posterior thyroid and two are located toward the inferior portion of the thyroid. Produces hormones (discussed in physiology).
Larynx	This is the region in the area of cervical 3 through cervical 6. This is the area that is the entrance to the trachea and esophagus. (discussed in detail in a later chapter).

Lymphatics	Many lymph nodes are located along the edges of the right and left internal jugular veins. 　　Most of the lymph from the cervical lymph nodes drains into the left subclavian vein. Lymph nodes are generally oval-shaped and around 1 cm in size or smaller. 　　Lymph nodes act as part of our immune system. Lymph nodes contain leukocytes that are involved in fighting infectious agents.
Trachea	To be discussed in detail in a later chapter.
Esophagus	To be discussed in detail in a later chapter.
Tonsils	To be discussed in detail in a later chapter.

Chapter 5:   The Upper Appendage Region

The upper appendage consists of four segments:

1. Shoulder (scapula): The shoulder (pectoral girdle) consists of the scapula and clavicle. The shoulder connects the torso to the upper appendage.

2. Arm (brachium): This articulates with the scapula and the forearm.

3. Forearm (antebrachium): This articulates with the humerus and the wrist.

4. Hand (manus): This is distal to the antebrachium and is composed of the wrist and digits and an opposable thumb.

5 A.   The entire skeleton consists of 206 individual bones. The appendicular skeleton, which consists of the pectoral girdle (shoulder), arms, pelvic girdle (hip), and legs, comprises 126 bones. This chapter only pertains to the upper appendicular skeleton, which is comprised of 64 bones.

5 B.   There are over 700 skeletal muscles of the human body. The following tables are designed to help you study the muscles of the arms. This course is not designed to identify all 700, however, we will cover a substantial amount. The study of the origin and insertion of muscles can be found in Chapter 10.

5C.   The best way to study the blood vessels is to put a drop of blood in a starting point and identify the vessels as the drop of blood flows through the arm. Examine figures in the textbook as you study the following tables. Keep in mind; the following tables were designed to simplify the study of the blood vessels. The main concept is; identify one blood vessel and then identify the next blood vessel in sequence regarding the flow of blood.

5D.   The nerves of the upper arm arise from the cervical plexus and the brachial plexus. You will notice that the plexus appears as a "tangled" mass of nerves. The word plexus means "braided." The nerves actually are not tangle but are organized in a special manner. The task at hand is to identify the parts of the plexus by separating them into an understandable manner.

Chapter 5A: The Skeleton

This chapter concentrates on the pectoral girdle, arm, wrist, and hand bones, which consist of 64 separate bones.

Upper Appendage Bones	
Scapula	2
Clavicle	2
Humerus	2
Radius	2
Ulna	2
Carpals	16 (8 per wrist)
Metacarpals	10 (5 per hand)
Phalanges	28 (14 per hand)
Total	**64**

While studying the structures in the table below, be sure to examine the figures in your textbook.

	Bone Structure	Description
1	Spinous process	This is a large, prominent ridge on the posterior side of the scapula. Sometimes just called the spine.
2	Acromion	This is a bulge located at the lateral edge of the spine of the scapula.
3	Supraspinous fossa	This is a depression immediately superior to the spine.
4	Infraspinous fossa	This is a depression immediately inferior to the spine.
5	Inferior angle	This is located at the most distal end of the scapula.
6	Superior angle	This is located at the most superior portion of the scapula.
7	Glenoid cavity	This is a depression located on the lateral edge nearest the acromion of the scapula.
8	Lateral border	This is the border of the scapula located in line with the glenoid cavity (axillary border).
9	Medial border	This is the border of the scapula nearest the spinal column (vertebral border).
10	Coracoid process	This is a bulge located near the glenoid cavity, anterior to the acromion.
11	Suprascapular notch	This is a rather prominent, anterior notch located between the superior angle and the coracoid process, nearest the coracoid process.
12	Subscapular fossa	This is the main portion of the complete anterior side of the scapula. The fossa is the depression that is close to the area of the suprascapular notch.

THE CLAVICLE

While studying the structures in the table below, be sure to examine the figures in your textbook.

	Bone Structure	Description
1	**Sternal end**	This is the medial end of the clavicle. It connects to the manubrium of the sternum.
2	**Acromial end**	This is the lateral end of the clavicle. It connects to the acromion of the scapula.
3	**Conoid tubercle**	This is a bulge on the inferior, posterior aspect of the clavicle nearest the acromial end.

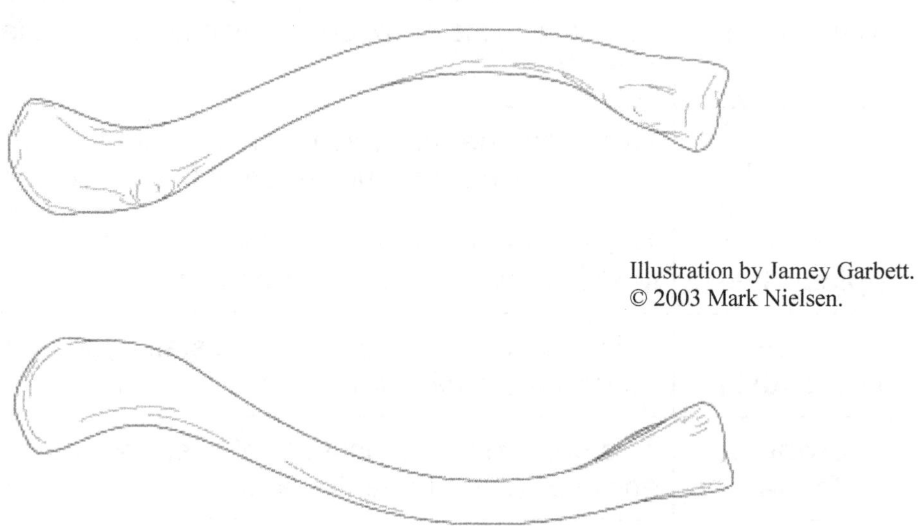

Illustration by Jamey Garbett.
© 2003 Mark Nielsen.

The table below identifies the structures of the humerus. While studying the contents of the table, be sure to examine the figures in your textbook.

	Bone Structure	Description
1	Head	This is the superior, rounded portion of the humerus.
2	Greater tubercle	This is a rather large bulge located lateral to the head.
3	Lesser tubercle	This is a smaller bulge located on the anterior aspect of the humerus nearest the head.
4	Intertubercular sulcus	This is a groove located between the greater tubercle and the lesser tubercle.
5	Deltoid tuberosity	This is a roughened area located a few centimeters inferior to the greater tubercle.
6	Capitulum	This is one of the condyles located at the distal end of the humerus. This rounded condyle is the most lateral of the two condyles.
7	Trochlea	This is another condyle located at the distal end of the humerus. This condyle is the most medial of the two condyles.
8	Medial epicondyle	This is a rather large bulge located on the distal, medial edge of the humerus, nearest the trochlea.
9	Lateral epicondyle	This is a bulge located on the distal, lateral edge of the humerus, nearest the capitulum.
10	Coronoid fossa	This depression is located between the medial and lateral epicondyles on the anterior side.
11	Olecranon fossa	This depression is located on the distal, posterior side of the humerus (posterior to the coronoid fossa).

THE ULNA

The two tables below identify the structures of the ulna and radius. While studying the contents of the tables, be sure to examine the figures in your textbook.

	Bone Structure	Description
1	Olecranon	This is the large, rounded, posterior bulge located at the proximal end of the ulna.
2	Trochlear notch	This is the huge notch or depression located at the proximal, anterior end of the ulna.
3	Coronoid process	This is a rim located at the most anterior edge of the trochlear notch.
4	Radial notch of the ulna	This is a shallow depression located lateral to the trochlear notch nearest the coronoid process.
5	Styloid process	This is a pointy process located at the distal end of the ulna.

THE RADIUS

	Bone Structure	Description
1	Head	This is the most proximal part of the radius. It is rounded and has a depression in the middle of it. It pivots on the capitulum of the humerus.
2	Radial tuberosity	This is a bulge located just a few centimeters distal to the head.
3	Dorsal radial tuberosity	This is a bumpy area located on the posterior side at the distal end.
4	Styloid process	This is a pointy process located at the distal and lateral end of the radius.

The table below identifies the bones and structures of the wrist. While studying the contents of the table, be sure to examine the figures in your textbook. Note, the descriptions are of an anterior view.

	Bone	Description
1	Capitate	This is the most central carpal bone in line with metacarpal III.
2	Hamate	This carpal is medial to the capitate.
3	Pisiform	This carpal is medial to the hamate. It is a small, rounded bone. It is attached to the triquetrum.
4	Triquetrum	Posterior to the pisiform is the triquetrum.
5	Lunate	This carpal is lateral to the triquetrum.
6	Scaphoid	This carpal is lateral to the lunate.
7	Trapezium	Articulating with metacarpal I is the trapezium.
8	Trapezoid	Medial to the trapezium is the trapezoid.
9	Metacarpals	The metacarpals are numbered beginning with the thumb side.
10	Digits	The digits are numbered beginning with the thumb. The thumb is digit I. Each digit consists of a proximal, middle, and distal phalanx except the thumb. The thumb consists of a proximal and a distal phalanx.

Articulations

This section concentrates on the ligaments that hold one bone to another, thereby creating the joints of the shoulder and the elbow.

The ligament names are rather scary because they are so long and consist of many syllables. However, break the name down and it usually consists of part of the name of one bone and part of the name of another bone or structure. While studying the following charts, be sure to examine the figures in your textbook.

Clavicle and Scapular Ligaments

	Ligament	Description
1	**Coracoclavicular ligament**	Consists of two parts: Trapezoid ligament: connects clavicle to coracoid process Conoid ligament: connects coracoid process to conoid tubercle.
2	**Acromioclavicular ligament**	Connects clavicle to acromion process.
3	**Coracoacromial ligament**	Connects coracoid process to acromial process
4	**Sternoclavicular ligament**	Connects the sternal end of the clavicle to the manubrium.
5	**Glenohumeral ligament**	Extends from the greater tubercle to the rim of the glenoid cavity

Bursa sac
Subdeltoid (subacromial): Cushions the proximal humerus when it is in the abducted position.

	Ligament	Description
1	**Ulnar collateral ligament**	Connects the medial epicondyle of the humerus to the ulna
2	**Radial collateral ligament**	Connects the lateral epicondyle of the humerus to the radius
3	**Annular ligament**	Connects the head of the radius to the ulna

Bursa sac
There is a bursa sac covering the olecranon process. This bursa sac prevents abrasion of the skin when the antebrachium is in the flexed position.

Below is some additional information regarding the skeleton of the upper appendage. Your instructor may add to this list.

1. Phalanx is a Latin term that means "line of soldiers."

2. You can easily palpate the following:
   a. Clavicle
   b. Greater tubercle
   c. Olecranon process
   d. Styloid process of the ulna
   e. Medial epicondyle of the humerus
   f. Lateral epicondyle of the humerus
   g. Spinous process of the scapula
   h. Medial border of the scapula
   i. Inferior border of the scapula

3. If you position the scapula so the glenoid cavity is right lateral and the spinous process is posterior, you have the right scapula.

4. If you position the humerus so the greater tubercle is left lateral and the olecranon fossa is posterior, you have the left humerus.

5. If you position the radius so the styloid process is right lateral and the dorsal radial tuberosity is posterior, you have the right radius.

6. If you position the ulna so the olecranon process is posterior and the radial notch of the ulna is left lateral, you have the left ulna.

7. Coracoid process is Latin that means "like a bird's beak."

8. The head of the humerus and the glenoid fossa create the ball-and-socket joint of the shoulder.

9. Glenoid comes from the Greek word, gleno, which means "socket."

10. The head of the humerus is the ball of the ball and socket joint of the shoulder. The head articulates with the glenoid cavity.

11. Huge muscles attach to the greater tubercle.

12. A tendon of the long head of the biceps brachii muscle passes through intertubercular sulcus to connect to the superior portion of the glenoid cavity.

13. A portion of the deltoid muscle attaches to the deltoid tuberosity.

14. Trochlea is Latin that means "like a spool." Examine the trochlea to see that, indeed, it looks like a spool (as in a spool of thread).

15. Notice that there is a notch between the medial epicondyle and the medial edge of the trochlea. The ulnar nerve passes through this area. When this nerve is hit, a tingly sensation is felt. Many refer to this as the "funny bone."

16. In the flexed position, the coronoid process of the ulna fits into the coronoid fossa of the humerus.

17. In the extended position, the olecranon process of the ulna fits into the olecranon fossa of the humerus

18. You can feel the spine of the scapula.

19. You can feel bumps at the lateral edge of your shoulder. These bumps are the combination of the acromial end of the clavicle and the acromion of the scapula.

20. You can feel the inferior angle of the scapula.

21. You can feel the medial border of the scapula. It is close to the spinal column.

22. The sternal end of the clavicle appears to be "squared off" a bit.

23. There are numerous ligaments associated with the sternal end and the manubrium.

24. The acromial end appears to be sort-of rounded and flattened.

25. There are numerous ligaments associated with the acromial end and the coracoid process.

26. There is a ligament that extends from the conoid tubercle to the coracoid process.

27. The olecranon process is our elbow.

28. The trochlear notch sort-of looks like an ice cream scoop from a side view.

29. The head of the radius pivots in the radial notch of the ulna.

30. The posterior side of the radius at the distal end is bumpy and the anterior side of the radius at the distal end is smooth.

31. The capitate is a columnar-shaped bone. This carpal articulates with metacarpal III.

32. The hamate has a hook. This carpal articulates with metacarpal IV and V.

33. The lunate articulates with a portion of the ulna and the radius.

34. The scaphoid articulates with the radius.

35. The trapezium is in line with the thumb. This carpal articulates with metacarpal I.

36. The trapezoid is actually a four-sided bone; but it appears to be "trapped" between the trapezium and the capitate. This carpal articulates with metacarpal II.

37. The metacarpals are a series of parallel bones you can feel on the back of your hand.

38. The digits are called phalanges. Each individual bone of a digit is called a phalanx.

Chapter 5B: The Muscles

This chapter concentrates on the skeletal muscles of the arms

MUSCLES OF THE BRACHIUM

	Muscle	Description
	Anterior Muscles of the Brachium	
1	**Biceps brachii**	There are two heads to the biceps brachii. There are two origins of these muscles but they merge together to form one insertion. **Short head**: this portion is medial. **Long head**: this portion is lateral.
2	**Brachialis**	This muscle is deep to the biceps brachii.
3	**Coracobrachialis**	This muscle is deep and medial to the short head of the biceps brachii.
	Posterior Muscles of the Brachium	
4	**Triceps brachii**	There are three heads to the triceps brachii. There are three origins of these muscles but they merge together to form one insertion. **Long head**: this portion is between the lateral head and the medial head. **Lateral head**: this portion is lateral. **Medial head**: this portion is medial and deep to the long head.

The best way to study the muscles is to begin with a landmark (a specific muscle) and then go medial to it or lateral to it, for example.

	Muscle	Description
	Anterior Muscles of the Antebrachium	
1	**Palmaris longus**	This muscle is in the center of the antebrachium and has a tendon that extends to the palm of the hand.
2	**Flexor digitorum superficialis**	Deep to the palmaris longus.
3	**Flexor carpi ulnaris**	Medial to the palmaris longus.
4	**Flexor carpi radialis**	Lateral to the palmaris longus.
5	**Pronator teres**	Lateral to the flexor carpi radialis. This muscle extends through the antecubital region.
6	**Brachioradialis**	Lateral to the pronator teres. This is the most lateral muscle of the antebrachium.
7	**Flexor pollicis longus**	This appears as a proximal oblique muscle near the carpal region on the lateral side.
8	**Pronator quadratus**	This is an transverse muscle that is distal to the flexor pollicis longus near the carpal region on the lateral side.
	Flexor retinaculum This is a transverse band of connective tissue surrounding the carpal region on the anterior side. This is not a muscle.	

MUSCLES OF THE ANTEBRACHIUM (continued)

	Muscle	Description
	Posterior Muscles of the Antebrachium	
9	**Extensor digitorum**	This muscle is in the center of the posterior antebrachium. It has tendons that branch to digits 2 through 5.
10	**Extensor digiti minimi**	Medial to the extensor digitorum.
11	**Extensor Carpi ulnaris**	Medial to the extensor digiti minimi.
12	**Anconeus**	Appears in the cubital region at the superior end of the carpi ulnaris and extensor digitorum.
13	**Abductor pollicis longus**	A muscle that is deep to the extensor digitorum and runs oblique to the thumb side.
14	**Extensor carpi radialis brevis**	Lateral to the extensor digitorum.
15	**Extensor carpi radialis longus**	Lateral to the extensor carpi radialis brevis.
16	**Extensor pollicis brevis**	A muscle that is deep to the extensor digitorum and runs oblique to the thumb side. It is distal to the abductor pollicis longus.

Extensor retinaculum
This is a transverse band of connective tissue in the carpal region. It is not a muscle.

HAND MUSCLES AND ROTATOR CUFF MUSCLES

The best way to study the muscles is to begin with a landmark (a specific muscle) and then go medial to it or lateral to it, for example. Be sure to keep the palm of the hand oriented correctly. There are four muscles we study on the palm of the hand. Two are associated with metatarsal V (**hypothenar** muscles) and two are associated with metatarsal I (**thenar** muscles).

There are four muscles that comprise the rotator cuff group. These muscles connect to either the greater tubercle or the lesser tubercle of the humerus.

	Muscle	Description
	Muscles of the Palm	
1	**Abductor digiti minimi**	The most medial muscle of the hand.
2	**Flexor digiti minimi**	Lateral to the abductor digiti minimi.
3	**Abductor pollicis brevis**	The most lateral muscle of the hand.
4	**Flexor pollicis brevis**	Medial to the abductor pollicis brevis.

ROTOR CUFF MUSCLES

	Muscle	Description
1	**Supraspinatus**	This muscle is superior to the spine of the scapula.
2	**Infraspinatus**	This muscle is inferior to the spine of the scapula.
3	**Teres minor**	This muscle is inferior to the distal end of the infraspinatus.
4	**Subscapularis**	This muscle is located in the subscapular fossa of the scapula.

THE MUSCLES: ADDITIONAL INFORMATION

Below is some additional information regarding the upper appendage muscles. Your instructor may add to this list.

1. When skeletal muscles contract, they pull. Generally, they pull toward the point of origin (discussed in a later chapter).

2. Skeletal muscles consist of striations and multiple nuclei.

3. Below is a list for better understanding of muscle terminology.

   a. Brevis: refers to short
   b. Longus: refers to long
   c. Bi: means two
   d. Tri: means three
   e. Carpi: means to grasp
   f. Teres: refers to small, cylindrical
   g. Pollicis: refers to pollex (thumb)
   h. Retinaculum: Latin for "like a halter"
   i. Digiti: refers to digits
   j. Minimi: refers to small

Chapter 5C: The Blood Vessels

The best way to study the blood vessels is to take a drop of blood and follow it through the vessels as it travels.

ARTERIES OF THE ARM

	Artery	Description
1	**Subclavian artery**	This artery arches across the shoulder area and goes under the clavicle.
2	**Axillary a**	The axillary artery goes through the axilla region.
3	**Brachial a**	The brachial artery is associated with the brachium and branches to form the radial and ulnar artery in the area of the antecubital region.
4	**Radial a / Ulnar a**	The radial artery runs along the radius (lateral antebrachium) and the ulnar artery runs along the ulna (medial antebrachium).
5	**Superficial palmar arch artery**	The radial artery and ulnar artery anastomose in the palm.

Veins of the Arm

This table describes the veins of the arms. Study the veins in the same manner as you studied the arteries. The veins return blood to the heart.

Deep Veins of the Arm

	Veins	Description
1	Superficial palmar arch vein	The veins anastomose in the palm of the hand.
2	Radial a / Ulnar v	These veins parallel their corresponding arteries and merge together in the antecubital region.
3	Brachial v	The brachial vein parallels the brachial a.
4	Axillary v	This vein is in the axilla region
5	Subclavian v	This vein lies under the clavicle and forms the left and right brachiocephalic veins.
6	Brachiocephalic v	The left and right brachiocephalic v merge to form the superior vena cava that enters into the right atrium of the heart.

VEINS OF THE ARM (continued)

This table describes other veins of the arms. Study the veins in the same manner as you studied the arteries. These veins are superficial veins in the arm

SUPERFICIAL VEINS OF THE ARM

	Veins	Description
1	Cephalic v	This vein runs on the lateral edge of the entire arm from the wrist area to the subclavian v.
2	Basilic v	This vein runs on the medial edge of the entire arm from the wrist area to the axillary v.
3	Median cubital v	Blood in the cephalic vein can merge over to the basilic v via the median cubital vein, which is located near the antecubital region.

Below is some additional information regarding the blood vessels of the upper appendage. Your instructor may add to this list.

1. The sequence of the flow of blood through the brachial artery is in this manner:

   Brachial artery to the radial artery **AND** ulnar artery.

2. The flow of blood through the brachial artery is **NOT** in this manner:

   Brachial artery to the radial artery and then to the ulnar artery.

3. Arteries carry blood away from the heart while veins carry blood toward the heart. It does not matter if the blood is oxygenated or deoxygenated.

4. Veins are commonly more superficial than arteries.

5. Veins have valves at various intervals to allow for the flow of blood only toward the heart.

Chapter 5D: The Nerves

The nerves of the upper arm arise from the cervical plexus and the brachial plexus. You will notice that the plexus appears as a "tangled" mass of nerves. The word plexus means "braided." The nerves actually are not tangle but are organized in a special manner. The task at hand is to identify the parts of the plexus by separating them into an understandable manner.

THE NERVES OF THE ARM

	Cervical Plexus	Nerves that emerge primarily from the cervical region.
1	Phrenic nerve	Emerges from the area of cervical 3 through 5. It extends inferiorly and parallels the sternum on both sides. It innervates the diaphragm muscle.

	Brachial plexus	Nerves that emerge from the lower cervical and upper thoracic (T1) region and extend to the brachial region.
1	Musculocutaneous nerve	This nerve emerges off the lateral cord and innervates the muscle and skin of the brachium.
2	Radial nerve	The radial nerve emerges off the posterior cord and innervates the muscles along the radius.
3	Ulnar nerve	The ulnar nerve emerges off the medial cord and innervates the muscles along the ulna and extends to digit 5.

Below is some additional information regarding the nerves of the upper appendage. Your instructor may add to this list.

1. The ulnar nerve passes through the groove area that is created by the olecranon process and the medial epicondyle.

2. Damage to the brachial plexus can occur when a person falls off a pommel horse (for example) and catches the pommel horse in the axilla region.

3. There are only four plexus regions.
    a. Cervical plexus
    b. Brachial plexus
    c. Lumbar plexus
    d. Sacral plexus

4. There is not a thoracic plexus.

Chapter 6:   The Lower Appendage Region

The lower appendage consists of five major parts or regions.

1. Gluteal region: This is the region between the torso and the lower limbs. It consists of the os coxa. The gluteal region will be discussed with the torso region.

2. Femoral region: This is the upper leg that articulates with the os coxa. It consists of the femur.

3. Patellar region: The patella partially protects the knee joint.

4. Leg region (crus): The entire lower leg is the crus. It consists of parallel bones; the tibia and fibula. Current wording in anatomy is to refer to the upper leg as the thigh and the lower leg as the "leg."

5. Ankle and foot: This consists of 7 tarsal bones, 5 metatarsals, and 5 digits. Digit number 1 is the great toe (hallux).

6 A.   The entire skeleton consists of 206 individual bones. This appendicular skeleton consists of the pelvic girdle (hip), femur, patella, tibia, fibula, ankle, and foot. This chapter only pertains to the lower appendicular skeleton, which is comprised of 62 bones.

6 B.   There are over 700 skeletal muscles of the human body. The following tables are designed to help you study the muscles of the hip and legs. This course is not designed to identify all 700 skeletal muscles; however, we will cover a substantial amount. The study of the origin and insertion of muscles can be found in Chapter 10.

6C.   The best way to study the blood vessels is to put a drop of blood in a starting point and identify the vessels as the drop of blood flows through the arm. Examine figures in the textbook as you study the following tables. Keep in mind; the following tables were designed to simplify the study of the blood vessels. The main concept is; identify one blood vessel and then identify the next blood vessel in sequence regarding the flow of blood.

6D.   The nerves of the leg arise from the lumbar plexus and the sacral plexus. You will notice that the plexus appears as a "tangled" mass of nerves. The word plexus means "braided." The nerves actually are not tangle but are organized in a special manner. The task at hand is to identify the parts of the plexus by separating them into an understandable manner.

Chapter 6A: The Skeleton

This chapter concentrates on the pelvic girdle, legs, ankle, and foot. The pelvic girdle consists of the hip, which is made of two os coxa bones. Each os coxa is made of the ilium, pubis, and ischium.

Upper Appendage Bones	
Os coxa	2
Femur	2
Patella	2
Tibia	2
Fibula	2
Tarsals	14 (7 per ankle)
Metatarsals	10 (5 per foot)
Phalanges	28 (14 per foot)
Total	**62**

While studying the structures in table below, be sure to examine the figures in your textbook.

	Bone or Bone Structure	Description
1	Ilium	This is the major portion of the os coxa.
2	Ischium	This is the distal, rounded, posterior portion of the os coxa. We sit on part of the ischium.
3	Pubis	This is the most anterior portion of the os coxa.
4	Acetabulum	This is the huge depression on the lateral side of the os coxa.
5	Obturator foramen	This is the huge hole located inferior to the acetabulum.
6	Iliac crest	This is the superior rim of the ilium.

7	**Anterior superior iliac spine**	This is a subtle bump on the anterior edge of the iliac crest.
8	**Anterior inferior iliac spine**	This is a subtle bump inferior to the anterior superior iliac spine.
9	**Posterior superior iliac spine**	This is a subtle bump on the posterior edge of the iliac crest.
10	**Posterior inferior iliac spine**	This is a subtle bump inferior to the posterior superior iliac spine.
11	**Greater sciatic notch**	This is a huge notch on the posterior side of the os coxa.
12	**Ischial spine**	This is a projection that is at the inferior aspect of the greater sciatic notch.

THE FEMUR

The table below describes the location of various femur structures. Examine the figures in your textbook while studying the table below.

	Bone or Bone Structure	Description
1	Head	This is the rounded portion of the femur that articulates with the acetabular fossa.
2	Fovea (Fovea capitis)	This is a depression in the center of the head of the femur.
3	Greater trochanter	Lateral to the head of the femur is a huge bulge.
4	Neck	Between the greater trochanter and the head is the neck of the femur.
5	Lesser trochanter	Inferior to the neck on the medial aspect of the femur is a small bulge called the lesser trochanter.
6	Medial condyle	This rounded process is located at the distal end on the medial aspect of the femur. It is best seen on the posterior side.
7	Lateral condyle	This rounded process is located at the distal end on the lateral aspect of the femur. It is best seen on the posterior side.
8	Intercondylar fossa	This is a depression located between the medial and lateral condyles.
9	Medial epicondyle	This is a bulge located medial to the medial condyle.

10	Lateral epicondyle	This is a bulge located lateral to the lateral condyle.
11	Intertrochanteric line	This is a small ridge extending from the greater trochanter to the lesser trochanter on the anterior side.
12	Intertrochanteric crest	This is a small ridge extending from the greater trochanter to the lesser trochanter on the posterior side.
13	Medial supracondylar line	This is a small ridge that angles over to the lateral epicondyle on the posterior side.
14	Lateral supracondylar line	This is a small ridge that angles over to the medial epicondyle on the posterior side.
15	Linea aspera	This is a small ridge that extends from the area of the lesser trochanter and splits to form the supracondylar lines.

THE TIBIA / FIBULA / PATELLA

The table below describes the location of various tibia and fibula structures. The tibia is the medial bone of the lower leg, and the fibula is the lateral bone of the lower leg. Examine the figures in your textbook while studying the table below.

Bone or Bone Structure		Description
		Tibia
1	**Intercondylar tubercles**	These are two bulges on the superior edge of the tibia. The intercondylar eminence is made of the intercondylar tubercles.
2	**Tibial tuberosity**	This is a bulge that is inferior to the patella.
3	**Anterior border**	This is a ridge that runs down the middle of the anterior tibia.
4	**Soleal line**	This is an oblique ridge located at the proximal end of the posterior tibia.
5	**Medial malleolus**	This is a bulge on the distal, medial end of the tibia.
		Fibula
1	**Head**	The head is at the proximal end and appears to be sort-of triangular in shape.
2	**Lateral malleolus**	This is a bulge on the distal end of the fibula.
		Patella
1	**Base**	The base is sort-of flat. It is the superior portion of the patella.
2	**Apex**	The apex is sort-of pointy at the inferior end of the patella.

THE ANKLE AND FOOT

The tables below identify the bones and structures of the ankle and foot. While studying the contents of the tables, be sure to examine the figures in your textbook.

THE ANKLE

1	Talus	The superior tarsal bone
2	Calcaneus	The posterior tarsal bone
3	Navicular	This tarsal is anterior to the talus.
4	Medial cuneiform	The three cuneiform bones are anterior to the navicular.
5	Intermediate cuneiform	
6	Lateral cuneiform	
7	Cuboid	The cuboid bone is anterior to the calcaneus and lateral to the lateral cuneiform.

THE FOOT

1	Metatarsals	The metatarsals are numbered beginning with the big toe moving lateral.
2	Digits	The digits are numbered beginning with the big toe. The big toe is digit I. Each digit consists of a proximal, middle, and distal phalanx except the big toe. The big toe consists of a proximal and a distal phalanx.

ARTICULATIONS

This section concentrates on the ligaments that hold one bone to another—
thereby creating the joints of the hip and the knee.

The ligament names are rather scary because they are so long and consist of
many syllables. However, break the name down and it usually consists of part of the
name of one bone and part of the name of another bone or structure. While studying
the following charts, be sure to examine the figures in your textbook.

LIGAMENTS OF THE HIP

	Ligament	Description
1	**Ligament of the head of the femur**	Also called the ligamentum teres. Connects the fovea capitis of the femoral head to the inside lining of the acetabulum.
2	**Iliofemoral ligament**	Connects from the intertrochanteric line to the acetabular rim.
3	**Pubofemoral ligament**	Connects from the greater trochanter area (on posterior side) to the pubis region (anterior side).
4	**Ischiofemoral ligament**	Connects from the greater trochanter area to the ischium.

	Ligament	Description
1	**Patellar ligament**	This is an extension of the rectus femoris tendon. It extends over the patella and connects to the tibial tuberosity.
2	**Fibular collateral ligament**	Formerly known as the lateral collateral ligament (LCL). Connects the lateral epicondyle of the femur to the head of the fibula.
3	**Tibial collateral ligament**	Formerly known as the medial collateral ligament (MCL). Connects the medial epicondyle of the femur to the medial, proximal edge of the tibia.
4	**Anterior cruciate ligament**	ACL: connects the intercondylar eminence of the tibia to the lateral side of the intercondylar fossa.
5	**Posterior cruciate ligament**	PCL: connects the intercondylar eminence of the tibia to the medial side of the intercondylar fossa.
6	**Medial and Lateral menisci**	These are pads of cartilage tissue that sit between the femoral condyles and the tibial faucets on the superior part of the tibia.

Bursa sac
Prepatellar bursa: This bursa sac lies anterior to the patella. It prevents abrasion from the skin when the lower leg is in the flexed position.

1. Acetabulum is Latin for "shallow vinegar cup."

2. The femur is the longest and heaviest bone of the body

3. You can easily palpate the following:
    a. Greater trochanter
    b. Ischial tuberosity
    c. Medial and lateral epicondyle of the femur
    d. Tibial tuberosity
    e. Medial malleolus
    f. Lateral malleolus
    g. Calcaneus
    h. Anterior border of the tibia

4. If you position the femur so the greater trochanter is right lateral and the femoral condyles are posterior, you have the right femur.

5. If you position the tibia so the tibial tuberosity is anterior and the medial malleolus is medial, you have the right tibia.

6. If you position the os coxa so the acetabulum is right lateral and the greater sciatic notch is posterior, you have the right os coxa.

7. The tibia articulates with the talus of the foot.

8. The angle between the pubic bones of the female (the angle inferior to the pubic symphysis) is larger than it is in males. This is to create a larger birthing area. This is referred to as the "subpubic angle."

9. The pleural of "pelvis" is "pelves."

10. There are eight carpal bones per wrist and seven tarsal bones per ankle.

11. The pubis bones are joined together by the **pubic symphysis**.

12. The head of the femur articulates with the acetabular fossa of the acetabulum.

13. Muscles pass through the obturator foramen

14. When you put your hands on your hips, you are putting your hands on the iliac crest.

15. The sciatic nerve passes through the greater sciatic notch.

16. The distance between the left ischial spine and the right ischial spine is the width of the pelvic inlet.

17. The ischium is pronounced,

    isk—ee—um   or   is—kee—um   but not   ish—ee—um.

18. The head of the femur fits into the acetabular fossa of the os coxa.

19. The fovea is also called the fovea capitis. The ligamentum teres extends from the fovea to the inside lining of the acetabulum.

20. Huge muscles attach to the greater trochanter.

21. You can feel the greater trochanter located lateral to your pants pocket area.

22. The femoral condyles articulate with the tibia in the popliteal region.

23. The ACL and PCL have attachments to the lining of the intercondylar fossa.

24. You can feel the medial condyle of the femur as a bulge medial to the patella area.

25. You can feel the lateral condyle as a bulge lateral to the patella area.

26. The ACL and PCL attach to the intercondylar tubercles.

27. You can feel the tibial tuberosity as a bulge slightly inferior to the patella.

28. The anterior border of the tibia can be felt as a sharp ridge on the anterior surface.

29. You can feel the medial malleolus as a bulge on the medial side of your ankle.

30. You can feel the lateral malleolus as a bulge on the lateral side of your ankle.

31. The patella is a sesamoid bone; it provides protection for the knee joint.

32. The calcaneus is our heel bone.

33. The metatarsals are parallel bones that make up the arch of the foot.

Chapter 6B: The Muscles

In this class, we will study at least 27 muscles of the lower appendage. The best way to study the muscles is to begin with a landmark (a specific muscle) and then go medial to it or lateral to it, etc.

THIGH MUSCLES

	Muscle	Description
	Anterior Muscles of the Femur	
1	**Rectus femoris**	This muscle is in the middle of the anterior femoral region and its tendon extends over the patella.
2	**Vastus lateralis**	Lateral to the rectus femoris
3	**Vastus medialis**	Medial to the rectus femoris
4	**Vastus intermedius**	This muscle is deep to the rectus femoris and is between the vastus medialis and vastus lateralis.
	Muscles 1, 2, 3, and 4 are collectively called the **quadriceps muscle group**.	
5	**Sartorius**	This muscle runs oblique from the lateral hip area to the medial side of the patella region and inserts on the tibial tuberosity.
6	**Gracilis**	The most medial muscle of the thigh

THIGH MUSCLES (continued)

The best way to study the muscles is to begin with a landmark (a specific muscle) and then go medial to it or lateral to it, etc.

	Muscle	Description
7	**Tensor fasciae latae**	The most lateral muscle of the thigh. This muscle has a long tendinous band that extends to the patella and inserts on the tibial tuberosity. This band is called the iliotibial tract.
8	**Adductor longus**	Anterior to the gracilis at the proximal end.
9	**Pectineus**	Lateral and superior to the adductor longus
10	**Iliopsoas**	Lateral and superior to the pectineus
	Posterior Muscles of the Femur	

11	**Biceps femoris**	There are two heads to the biceps femoris.
		    Long head: Posterior, lateral thigh muscle.
		    Short head: Deep to the long head.

12	**Semitendinosus**	This muscle is medial to the biceps femoris long head.
13	**Semimembranosus**	This muscle is deep to the semitendinosus.
	Muscles 11, 12, and 13 are collectively called the **hamstring muscle group**.	
14	**Adductor magnus**	This muscle appears between the semitendinosus and the gracilis. It is posterior to the gracilis.

GLUTEAL MUSCLES

Use your textbook to examine figures of the muscles of the gluteal region.

	Muscle	Description
		Muscles of the Gluteal Region
1	**Gluteus maximus**	This is the superficial gluteal muscle.
2	**Gluteus medius**	This muscle is deep to the gluteus maximus.
3	**Gluteus minimus**	This muscle is deep to the gluteus medius.
4	**Piriformis**	This muscle is inferior to the gluteus minimus.
5	**Gemellus superior**	This muscle is inferior to the piriformis.
6	**Obturator internus**	This muscle is inferior to the gemellus superior. This muscle passes through the obturator foramen.
7	**Gemellus inferior**	This muscle is inferior to the obturator internus.
8	**Quadratus femoris**	This muscle is inferior to the gemellus inferior.

Muscles 2 through 8 insert on the greater trochanter.

The gluteus maximus forms a tendon sheath with the tensor fasciae latae muscle, which inserts on the tibialis anterior in the area just inferior to the patella. This tendon sheath is the **iliotibial band** (tract).

Muscles 4 through 8 are known as the **lateral rotator group**.

The best way to study the muscles is to begin with a landmark (a specific muscle) and then go medial to it or lateral to it, etc.

		Posterior Muscles of the Lower Leg
1	**Gastrocnemius**	There are two heads to the gastrocnemius. Lateral head Medial head These muscles merge to form a long tendon that attaches to the calcaneus (calcaneal tendon).
2	**Soleus**	Deep to the gastrocnemius
3	**Popliteus**	This muscle is in the popliteal area and runs oblique from lateral to medial. This muscle is deep to the gastrocnemius.
4	**Plantaris**	This muscle is also in the popliteal area, but it has a tendon that runs from the popliteal area all the way to the foot. This muscle is also deep to the gastrocnemius.
		Anterior Muscles of the Lower Leg
5	**Tibialis anterior**	This muscle is actually a bit lateral to the anterior border tibia.
6	**Fibularis longus and fibularis brevis**	These two muscles are the most lateral muscle of the lower leg.
7	**Extensor digitorum longus**	This muscle is between the tibialis anterior and fibularis longus.

HELPFUL HINTS FOR IDENTIFYING A FEW SELECT MUSCLES

Use other figures in your textbook to help you identify the muscles in the table below.

<table>
<tr><td colspan="2" align="center">**Look at an Anterior View of the Thigh**</td></tr>
<tr><td colspan="2">Find the sartorius and the gracilis.
    Between the sartorius and the gracilis are several muscles.
        Begin with the gracilis and go anterior to find the adductor longus.
            Go anteriorly-lateral from the adductor longus to find the pectineus.
            Go anteriorly-lateral from the pectineus to find the iliopsoas.</td></tr>
<tr><td colspan="2" align="center">**Look at a Medial View of the Thigh**</td></tr>
<tr><td colspan="2">Find the gracilis.
    Anterior to the gracilis is the adductor longus.
    Posterior to the gracilis is the adductor magnus.</td></tr>
<tr><td colspan="2" align="center">**Look at a Medial View of the Lower Leg in the Ankle Area**</td></tr>
<tr><td>Find the tendon of the **T**ibialis posterior.
    Go posterior to find the tendon of the flexor **D**igitorum longus.
        Go posterior to find an **A**rtery.
            Go posterior to find a **N**erve.
                Go posterior to find the tendon of the flexor **H**allucis longus.</td><td>**T**om
Dick
an (and)

Harry</td></tr>
</table>

MUSCLES OF THE FOOT

Use your textbook to examine figures of the muscles of the foot.

	Muscle	Description
		Muscles of the Foot
1	**Flexor digitorum brevis**	This is a large muscle in the middle of the bottom of the foot. Its tendons attach to digits 1 through 5.
2	**Abductor digiti minimi**	This is a large muscle that is lateral to the flexor digitorum brevis.
3	**Abductor hallucis**	This is a large muscle that is medial to the flexor digitorum brevis.

MUSCLES:
ADDITIONAL INFORMATION

Below is some additional information regarding the muscles of the lower appendage. Your instructor may add to this list.

1. Below is a list for better understanding of muscle terminology:
    a. Rectus: refers to straight
    b. Vastus: refers to covering a large area
    c. Sartorius comes from Latin, sartor, that means, "tailor."
    d. Gracilis is Latin that means, "slender."
    e. Magnus: in reference to large
    f. Soleus: in reference to a flat muscle.
    g. Gastrocnemius: gastro is in reference to stomach or belly. Nemius comes from the Latin, kneme, which means leg. Therefore, this muscle is so named because it refers to the belly of the leg (bulge on the posterior lower leg).
    h. Hallucis: refers the hallux.

2. The sartorius muscle is named in reference to tailors. In early days, a tailor would cross their leg in such a manner to create a flat table so they could sit and sew fabric.

3. The sartorius is our "leg crossing muscle."

4. The iliopsoas muscle (the "p" is silent) is made of two muscles; the iliacus and the psoas muscles.

Chapter 6C: The Blood Vessels

The best way to study the blood vessels is to put a drop of blood in a starting point and identify the vessels as the drop of blood flows through the lower appendage. Examine figures in the textbook as you study the following tables. Keep in mind; the following tables were designed to simplify the study of the blood vessels. The main concept is; identify one blood vessel and then identify the next blood vessel in sequence regarding the flow of blood.

THE ARTERIES OF THE LEG

	Artery	Description
1	**Common iliac artery**	Emerges from the descending aorta (abdominal aorta). Branches to form the external iliac a and the internal iliac a.
2	**External iliac a**	Forms the femoral a.
3	**Internal iliac a**	Branch off the common iliac that runs deep into the pelvis.
4	**Femoral a**	Runs the length of the femur and forms the popliteal a in the popliteal region.
5	**Popliteal a**	Branches to form the anterior and posterior tibial a.
5	**Anterior / Posterior tibial a**	The anterior tibial a is on the anterior aspect of the tibia. The posterior tibial a is on the posterior portion of the tibia and has a branch that forms the fibular a.

VEINS OF THE LEGS

This table describes the veins of the legs. Study the veins in the same manner as you studied the arteries. The veins return blood to the heart.

	Veins	Description
1	Anterior / Posterior tibial veins	The anterior and posterior tibial v will merge at the location of the popliteal v.
2	Fibular v	The fibular v joins the posterior tibial v.
3	Popliteal v	Forms the femoral v.
4	Femoral v	Forms the external iliac v.
5	External iliac v	Forms the common iliac v.
6	Common iliac v	The right and left common iliac veins join to form the inferior vena cava that leads to the right atrium of the heart.
7	Great saphenous v	Extends from the foot region and runs along the medial side of the leg and merges with the femoral v just slightly inferior to the junction of the femoral v and external iliac v.

THE BLOOD VESSELS: ADDITIONAL INFORMATION

Below is some additional information regarding the blood vessels of the lower appendage. Your instructor may add to this list.

1. The sequence of the flow of blood through the femoral artery is in this manner:

    Femoral artery to the popliteal artery to the anterior **AND** posterior tibial arteries

2. The flow of blood through the femoral artery is **NOT** in this manner:

    Femoral artery to the popliteal artery to the anterior tibial artery and then to the posterior tibial artery.

3. The great saphenous vein is medial to the femoral vein.

Chapter 6D: The Nerves

The nerves of the leg arise from the lumbar plexus and the sacral plexus. You will notice that the plexus appears as a "tangled" mass of nerves. The word plexus means "braided." The nerves actually are not tangle but are organized in a special manner. The task at hand is to identify the parts of the plexus by separating them into an understandable manner.

THE NERVES

1	**Lumbar plexus**	Nerves that emerge primarily from the lower back region. A major nerve arising from this plexus is the femoral nerve This nerve innervates the sartorius and the quadriceps
2	**Sacral plexus**	These nerves emerge from the lower back and the upper sacral region. A major nerve arising from this plexus is the sciatic nerve. This nerve innervates the hamstring muscles.

Below is some additional information regarding the nerves of the lower appendage. Your instructor may add to this list.

1. When a person lands real hard on their gluteal region, they might damage the lumbar or sacral plexus, which will then affect the nerves going to the leg muscles.

Chapter 7:   The Torso Region

The torso consists of the thoracic region and the abdominopelvic region. The torso is that part of the human body that excludes the head and limbs. We will examine different "sections" of the torso, which include the following:

1. Thoracic region
    a. Heart
    b. Thymus gland
    c. Lungs

2. Abdominal region
    a. Digestive system
    b. Liver
    c. Spleen
    d. Pancreas
    e. (kidneys are discussed in a later chapter)

7 A.   The skeletal portion of the torso will include the study of the ribs, sternum, and the vertebrae.

7 B.   The muscles in this chapter will include thoracic and abdominal muscles. Other muscles studied are the "breathing" muscles and the abdominal muscles.

7 C.	The study of blood in this chapter consists of two parts. The first part is the study of the heart, which includes the heart structures and the flow of blood through the heart. The second part includes the study of the blood vessels associated with the thoracic and abdominal regions.

7 D.	The study of the nerves of the torso region includes the nerve conduction system of the heart. Another major aspect of this chapter is the study of the spinal cord and peripheral nerves, which includes the sympathetic and parasympathetic systems.

7 E.	The torso has more divisions or regions than the other parts of the body. Therefore, this section (7 E) examines the structure of the lungs.

7 F.	Another section to be studied within the torso region is the digestive system. While studying this section, you are exposed to a little bit of digestive physiology.

Chapter 7A: The Ribs and Vertebrae

The thoracic region consists of the sternum and ribs and the vertebral column. The vertebral column consists of the vertebrae, sacrum, and coccyx. The table below lists the various bones and bone structures of the thoracic region. While studying this table, examine the pictures in your textbook.

The Ribs and Vertebrae	
Sternum	1
Ribs	24 (12 pair)
Vertebrae	24
Sacrum	1
Coccyx	1
Total	**51**

	Bone or Bone Structure	Description
1	Manubrium	This is the first part (superior part) of the sternum.
2	Body	This is the main part of the sternum. It is immediately inferior to the manubrium.
3	Xiphoid	This is the "pointy" part that is inferior to the body of the sternum.
4	Jugular notch	This is the depression at the superior edge of the manubrium.

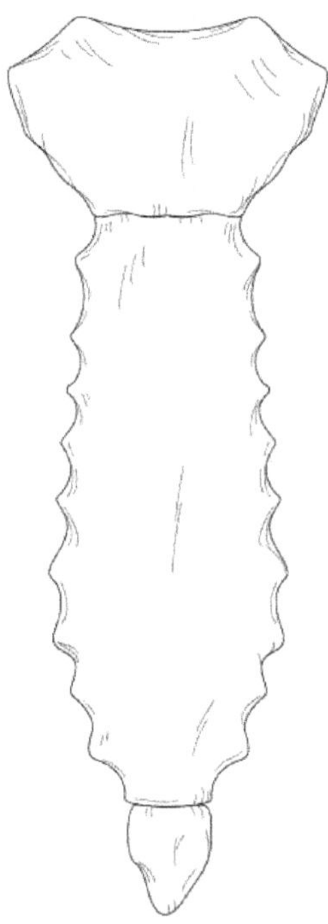

Illustration by Jamey Garbett.
© 2003 Mark Nielsen.

THE RIBS

The table below depicts the variety of classifications of the ribs. Refer to a picture of the thoracic cage with ribs attached while studying the table below.

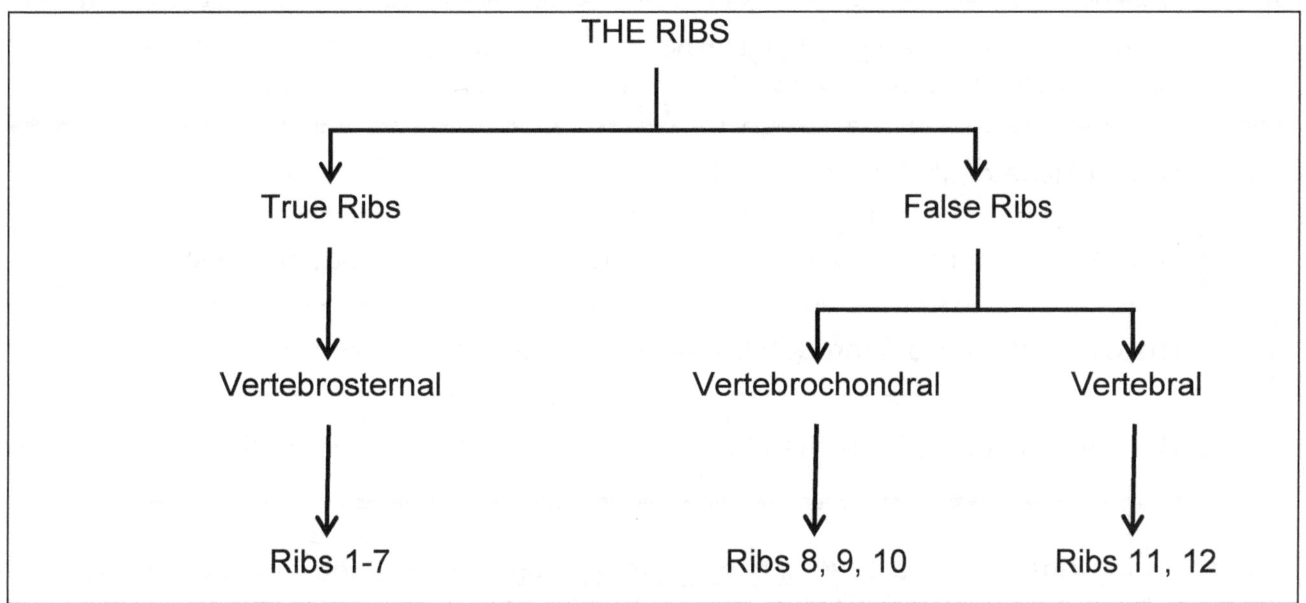

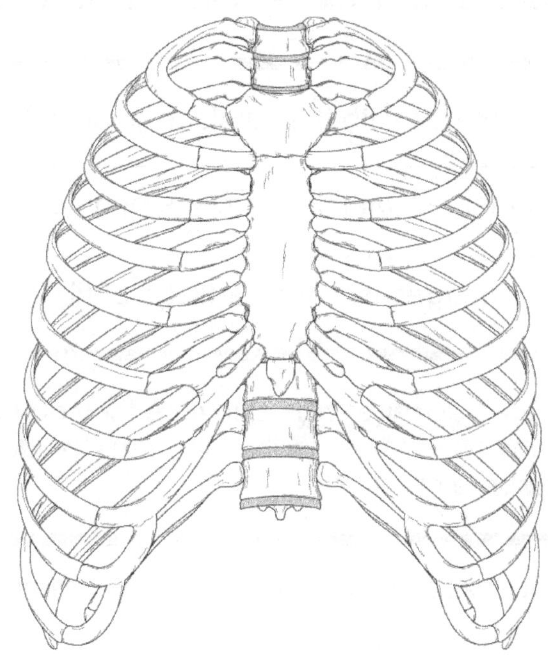

Illustration by Jamey Garbett.
© 2003 Mark Nielsen.

Rib number	Description
	The following ribs (1–7) are **vertebrosternal ribs** because the cartilage of those ribs has a direct attachment to some part of the sternum (hence the term "sternal").
1	The cartilage of rib 1 attaches to the manubrium.
2	The cartilage of rib 2 attaches to the manubrium and the body of the sternum.
3, 4, 5, 6	The cartilage of ribs 3 through 6 attaches to the body of the sternum.
7	The cartilage of rib 7 attaches to the body of the sternum and partially to the xiphoid.
	The following ribs (8–10) are **vertebrochondral ribs** because the cartilage of those ribs does not have a direct attachment to some part of the sternum. Their cartilage merges with the cartilage of the rib superior to them (hence "chondral" for cartilage).
8	The cartilage of rib 8 merges with the cartilage of rib 7.
9	The cartilage of rib 9 merges with the cartilage of rib 8.
10	The cartilage of rib 10 merges with the cartilage of rib 9.
	The following ribs (11–12) are **vertebral ribs** because they do not have any anterior cartilage and do not have any attachment to the sternum (hence "vertebral," referring to their attachment to the vertebrae only).
11 12	Ribs 11 and 12 do not have any attachment to the sternum.

THE VERTEBRAE

There are 26 bones that make up the entire vertebral column. Twenty-four bones are individual vertebrae. The sacrum and coccyx make up the other two vertebral column bones. Study the following table while examining the figures in your textbook.

		Description
		7 Cervical Vertebrae
1		Cervical number 1 is the **atlas** (C_1). The skull articulates with this vertebra.
2		Cervical number 2 is the **axis** (C_2). The atlas pivots on the axis.
3		The cervical vertebrae (C_1 through C_7) form an anterior curve of the spinal column.
4		The cervical vertebrae support the weight of the head.
		12 Thoracic Vertebrae
5		All 12 thoracic vertebrae (T_1 through T_{12}) have a pair of ribs attached to them.
6		There are 12 pairs of ribs in both sexes (24 total ribs).
7		The thoracic vertebrae form a posterior curve on the spinal column.
		5 Lumbar Vertebrae
8		The lumbar vertebrae form an anterior curve on the spinal column.
9		The lumbar vertebrae support the weight of the entire upper body.
		Sacrum and Coccyx
10		The sacrum is made of 5 vertebrae that fuse together by age 25. The sacrum forms a posterior curve on the spinal column. The coccyx is made of three to five fused vertebrae.

THE VERTEBRAL STRUCTURES

While studying the vertebral structures, be sure to examine the figures in your textbook. Most of the structures are seen easily on a thoracic vertebra.

	Bone Structure	Description
1	Body	This is the solid portion of the vertebra. It is an anterior structure when positioned in the body.
2	Spinous process	This is the part of the vertebra that is pointing posterior.
3	Vertebral foramen	The foramen located between the spinous process and the body. The spinal cord passes through this foramen.
4	Transverse process	These extend laterally to the vertebral foramen.
5	Lamina	This is the curved area between the spinous process and the transverse process.
6	Pedicle	This is the area between the body and the transverse process.
7	Dens	Only vertebra number 2 has a dens. It is an anterior projection on the axis.
8	Transverse foramen	Only cervical vertebrae have transverse foramina. These are the foramina associated with the transverse processes. The vertebral artery passes through these foramina.

The Vertebral Curvatures

Physicians examine the various curvatures of the vertebral column. The table below gives a brief description of the curves.

	Curvature	Description
1	**Cervical curve**	From a lateral view, the cervical curve is an anterior curve.
2	**Thoracic curve**	From a lateral view, the thoracic curve is a posterior curve.
3	**Lumbar curve**	From a lateral view, the lumbar curve is an anterior curve.
4	**Sacral curve**	From a lateral view, the sacral curve is a posterior curve.
Kyphosis: An exaggerated thoracic curve giving a "hump-back" appearance. **Lordosis**: An exaggerated lumbar curve giving a "sway-back" appearance.		
5	From a posterior view, the vertebral column is supposed to be straight.	
Scoliosis: An exaggerated lateral curve (posterior view).		

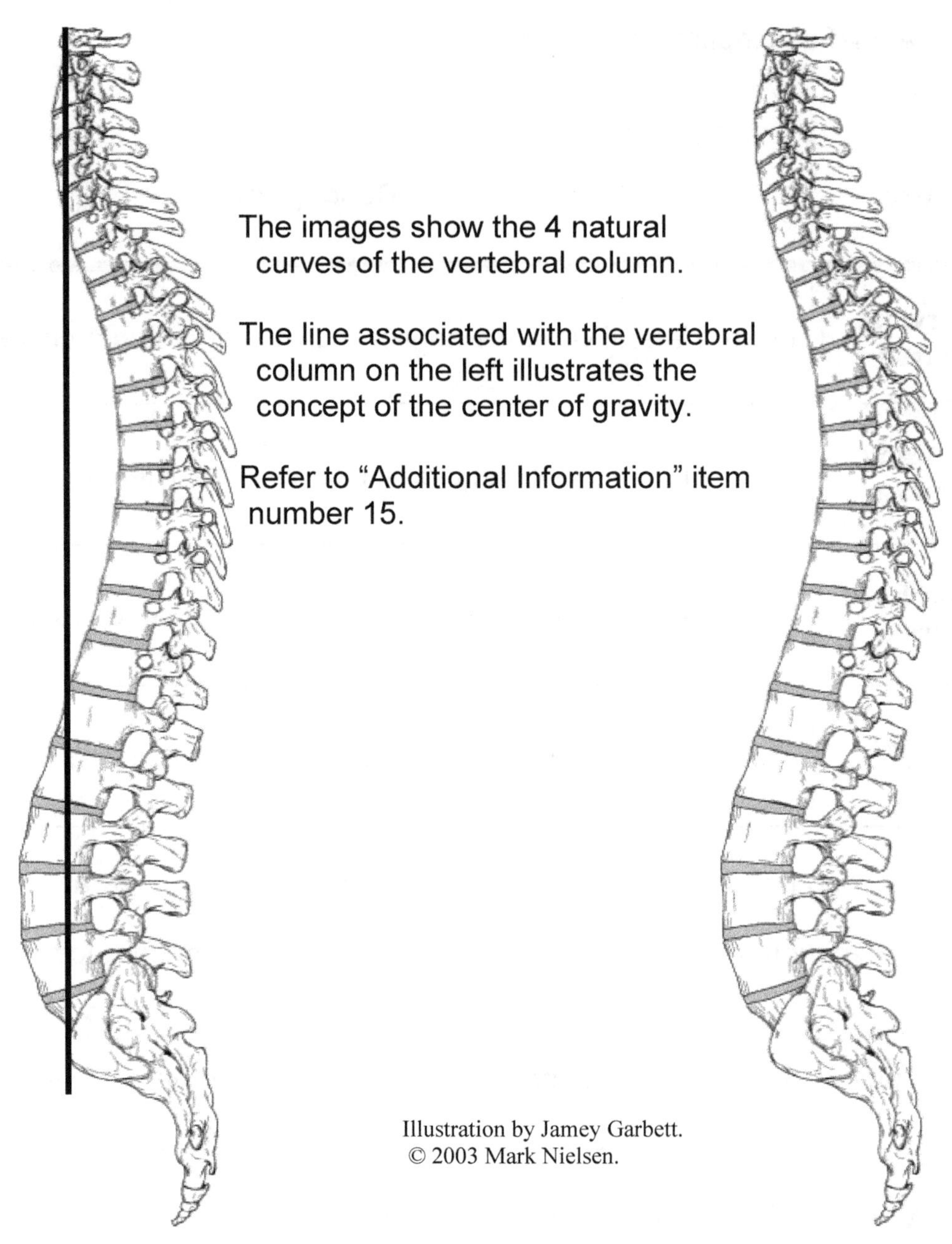

The images show the 4 natural curves of the vertebral column.

The line associated with the vertebral column on the left illustrates the concept of the center of gravity.

Refer to "Additional Information" item number 15.

Illustration by Jamey Garbett.
© 2003 Mark Nielsen.

THE RIBS AND VERTEBRAE: ADDITIONAL INFORMATION

Below is some additional information regarding the bones of the torso region. Your instructor may add to this list.

1. Only the thoracic vertebrae have ribs attached to them.

2. The atlas vertebra has facets for the attachment to the occipital condyles of the skull.

3. There are ligaments that wrap around the dens to help anchor the atlas in position.

4. The dens was formerly known as the odontoid process. Odontoid and dens are Latin for "like a tooth."

5. The skeleton is made of the axial and appendicular portions.

    a. The axial portion comprises the skull, vertebrae, ribs, and sternum.
    b. The appendicular portion comprises the pectoral girdle, pelvic girdle, and appendages.

        i. The pectoral girdle comprises the clavicle and the scapula.
        ii. The pelvic girdle comprises the os coxa.

6. The vertebral foramen is the large hole that the spinal cord passes through.

7. In males, the coccyx curves anteriorly and in females the coccyx projects mostly inferiorly. This allows for a larger birth canal region in females.

8. The approximately 4–10% of the population has a sternal foramen. This is a hole in the body of the sternum.

    a. During development, the body of the sternum is in two longitudinal parts. These two parts normally fuse together to form a solid body.

    b. If those two longitudinal parts of the sternum do not fuse properly, a hole will appear. Forensic scientists need to be clear on this foramen to avoid mistaking it for a bullet wound.

9. Cartilage that is on the anterior portion of the ribs is called **costal cartilage**.

10. The ribs have two points of attachment to the vertebrae. One point is on the superior edge of the body of one vertebra and the other point of attachment is on the inferior edge of the body of the vertebra superior to it.

11. Ribs have another point of attachment. They attach to a portion of each transverse process of the vertebrae.

12. All ribs have an attachment to the thoracic vertebrae. There are 12 thoracic vertebrae, therefore 12 pairs of ribs.

13. It is abnormal and potentially dangerous to have a cervical rib or a lumbar rib.

14. The vertebral arch is made of the lamina and pedicle.

15. The cervical vertebrae support the weight of the head.
    The lumbar vertebrae support the weight of the entire torso.
    The thoracic ribs only support the ribs.

Chapter 7B: The Torso Muscles

Use your textbook to examine figures of the muscles of the abdomen.

Description of the Abdominal Muscles

Begin with the **external oblique**. This muscle extends from the latissimus dorsi (muscle of the back) and wraps around the abdomen, forming a sheath that covers the anterior portion of the rectus abdominis muscles.

Deep to the external oblique is the **internal oblique**. This muscle extends from the latissimus dorsi area and wraps around the abdomen, forming a sheath that splits so part of the sheath covers the anterior portion of the rectus abdominis and part of the sheath covers the posterior portion of the rectus abdominis.

Deep to the external oblique is the **transversus abdominis**. This muscle extends from the latissimus dorsi area and warps around the abdomen, forming a sheath that covers the posterior portion of the rectus abdominis muscles.

The **rectus abdominis** muscles are the anterior muscles of the abdomen that form two vertical columns. These muscles are segmented and are ensheathed in the **rectus sheath**.

Each segment of the rectus abdominis muscles consists of **tendinous intersections**.

The sheaths from the left muscles (mentioned above) and the right muscles (mentioned above) join together on the anterior side of the abdomen to form the **linea alba**.

Deep to the transversus abdominis is the parietal peritoneum of the abdominal cavity.

Use your textbook to examine figures of the muscles of the torso.

	Muscle	Description
1	**Pectoralis major**	Major muscle of the thoracic region
2	**Deltoid**	This is the shoulder muscle. It extends from the lateral clavicular region to the deltoid tuberosity.
3	**Trapezius**	This is the upper-back muscle. It extends to the lumbar area and across the shoulder to the clavicle and "up" the neck to the occipital region of the skull.
4	**Rhomboid**	The rhomboid muscles (major and minor) are deep to the trapezius.
5	**Supraspinatus**	This is deep to the trapezius and the deltoid. It is superior to the spine of the scapula.
6	**Infraspinatus**	This is deep to the trapezius and the deltoid. It is inferior to the spine of the scapula.
7	**Teres**	The teres (major and minor) are deep to the trapezius and deltoid. They are inferior to the infraspinatus of the scapula.
8	**Latissimus dorsi**	This is the lower-back muscle covering most of the lumbar region. It curves around and inserts on the floor of the intertubercular sulcus.
9	**Erector spinae**	This is a group of three muscles that are deep to the latissimus dorsi and trapezius. **Spinalis thoracis**: nearest the spinal column. **Longissimus thoracis**: lateral to the spinalis thoracis. **Iliocostalis thoracis**: lateral to the longissimus thoracis.
10	**Subscapularis**	This muscle covers the anterior surface of the body of the scapula.

Below is some additional information regarding the muscles of the torso region. Your instructor may add to this list.

1. Below is a list for better understanding of muscle terminology.

    a. Supraspinatus: above the spine of the scapula

    b. Infraspinatus: below the spine of the scapula

    c. Latissimus comes from Latin that means the widest.

Chapter 7C$_1$: The Heart

 In order to study the heart, one must first become oriented with the position of the heart. Become familiar with the anterior and posterior portions: this is necessary in order to understand the internal components of the heart. Examine figures of the heart in your textbook while studying the table below.

THE HEART...EXTERNAL VIEW

	Heart Structure	Description
1	**Apex**	The apex of the heart angles to the left of the midline.
2	**Inferior margin**	The inferior margin of the heart rests on the diaphragm muscle.
3	**Anterior interventricular sulcus**	This is a sulcus that contains the anterior interventricular artery (coronary artery). It descends the anterior portion of the heart and angles to the right of the apex.
4	**Posterior interventricular sulcus**	This is a sulcus that contains the posterior interventricular artery. It descends the posterior portion of the heart and goes straight to the apex.

Based on the position of the sulcus, you can determine if you are looking at the anterior aspect of the heart or the posterior aspect.
Based on determining if you are looking at the anterior portion of the heart, you can determine the right and left of the heart (keep in mind the anatomical position).
The heart is made of 4 chambers: two superior atria and two inferior ventricles.

While looking at the external view of the heart, study the coronary vessels.

	Coronary Vessels	Description
1	**Right coronary artery**	Branches off the base of the ascending aorta and follows a sulcus that is inferior to the right atrium. It circles around the heart to the posterior side to form the **posterior interventricular artery**.
2	**Left coronary artery**	Branches off the base of the ascending aorta and goes to the left a few centimeters before branching again. Branches to form the **anterior interventricular artery** and the **circumflex artery**.

The circumflex artery follows a sulcus that is inferior to the left atrium of the heart. It then circles around the left side of the heart to the posterior side and branches many times.

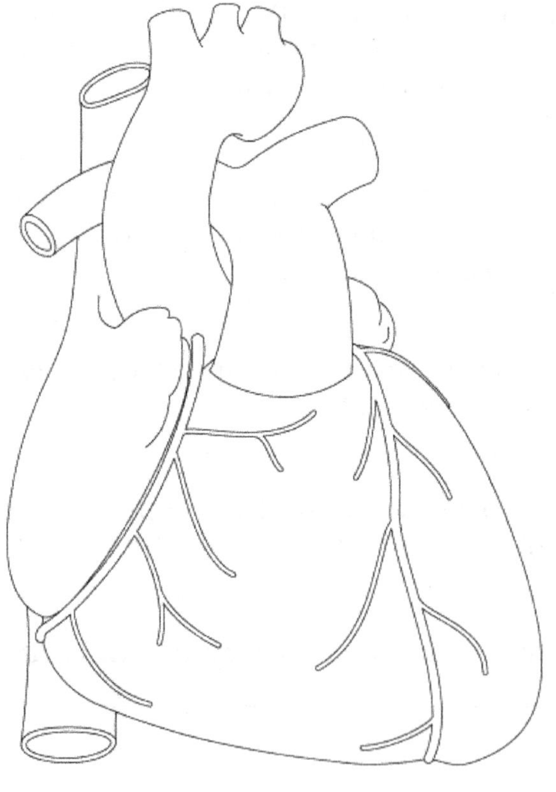

Illustrations by Jamey Garbett.
©2003 Mark Nielsen

THE HEART…INTERNAL VIEW

Look at the figures in your textbook to view the internal compartments of the heart. The table below describes many of the internal components.

	Heart Structures	Description
1	**Tricuspid valve**	Atrioventricular valve located in the right atrium that opens into the right ventricle. It is made of three cusps.
2	**Chordae tendineae**	Ligament-like structures that attach an atrioventricular valve to a papillary muscle.
3	**Papillary muscle**	Special muscles located on the inside lining of the ventricles and are attached to the atrioventricular valves via the chordae tendineae.
4	**Moderator band**	A muscular band that is found only in the right ventricle and extends from one wall of the ventricle to the other wall of the ventricle.
5	**Pulmonary valve**	A valve in the right ventricle that opens into the pulmonary trunk.
6	**Trabeculae carneae**	These are muscular structures located in both ventricles.
7	**Pectinate muscles**	These are muscular structures located mostly in the right atrium. They are less pronounced, if at all visible, in the left atrium.
8	**Bicuspid valve**	Atrioventricular valve located in the left atrium that opens into the left ventricle. This valve is also called the mitral valve. It is made of two cusps. Its real anatomical name is: valvula bicuspidalis.
9	**Aortic valve**	A valve located in the left ventricle that opens into the ascending aorta

10	**Interventricular septum**	Muscular septum that separates the left ventricle from the right ventricle
11		The wall of the left ventricle is thicker than the wall of the right ventricle. This makes the left side of the heart a stronger pump than the right side.
12		The cardiac cells (studied several chapters ago) are found in the walls of the heart.
13		The walls of the heart are made of three linings. **Endocardium**: The inside lining of the heart. **Myocardium**: The main muscular portion of the heart. **Epicardium**: The outside lining of the heart.

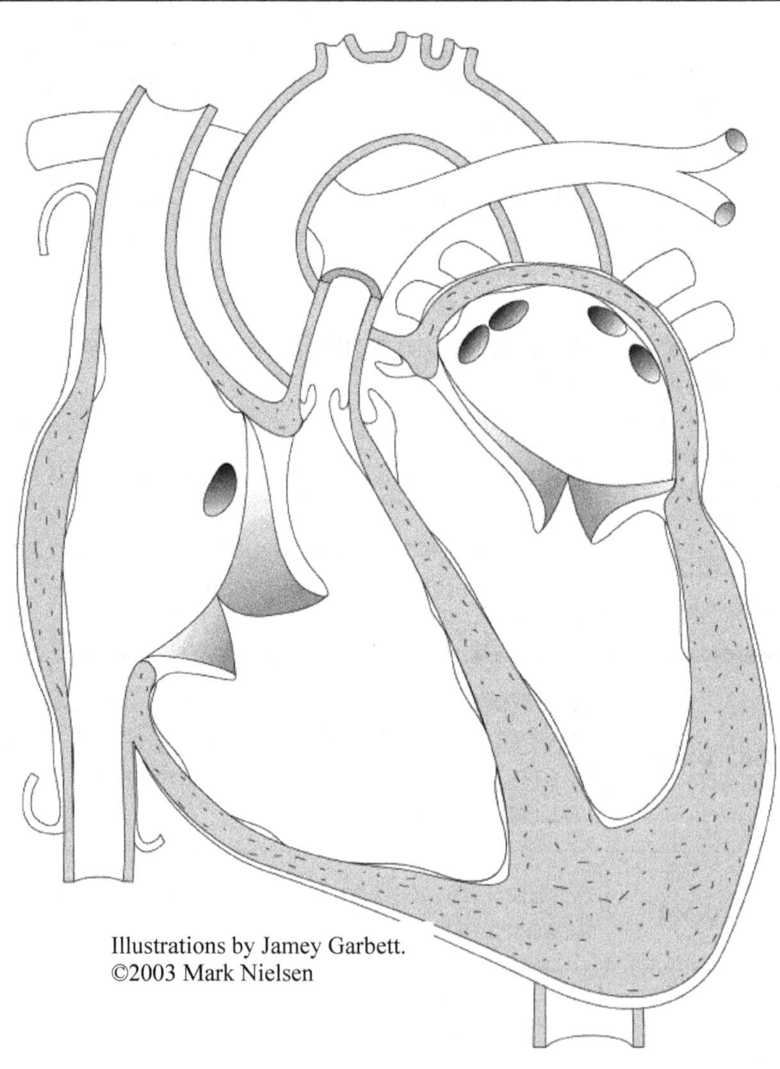

Illustrations by Jamey Garbett.
©2003 Mark Nielsen

CIRCULATION THROUGH THE HEART

The best way to study the heart is to put a drop of blood in the right atrium and follow it through the heart, out to the body, and back to the right atrium.

	Blood Flow through the Heart
1	Right atrium
2	Through the tricuspid valve
3	Into the right ventricle
4	Through the pulmonary valve (pulmonary semilunar valve / pulmonic valve)
5	Into the pulmonary trunk
6	Into the left and right pulmonary arteries
7	To the lungs to pick up oxygen (blood becomes oxygenated) and drop off carbon dioxide to be exhaled.
8	Into the left and right pulmonary veins
9	Enters into the left atrium
10	Passes through the bicuspid valve (mitral valve)
11	Into the left ventricle
12	Through the aortic valve (aortic semilunar valve)
13	Into the ascending aorta on its way to all body parts

The blood now has to return to the heart after dropping off oxygen at the body's tissues and picking up carbon dioxide.

	Blood Flow Back to the Heart
14	Blood from the lower extremities ultimately enters into the inferior vena cava (IVC) and enters into the right atrium.
15	Blood from the upper extremities ultimately enters into the superior vena cava (SVC) and the right atrium.

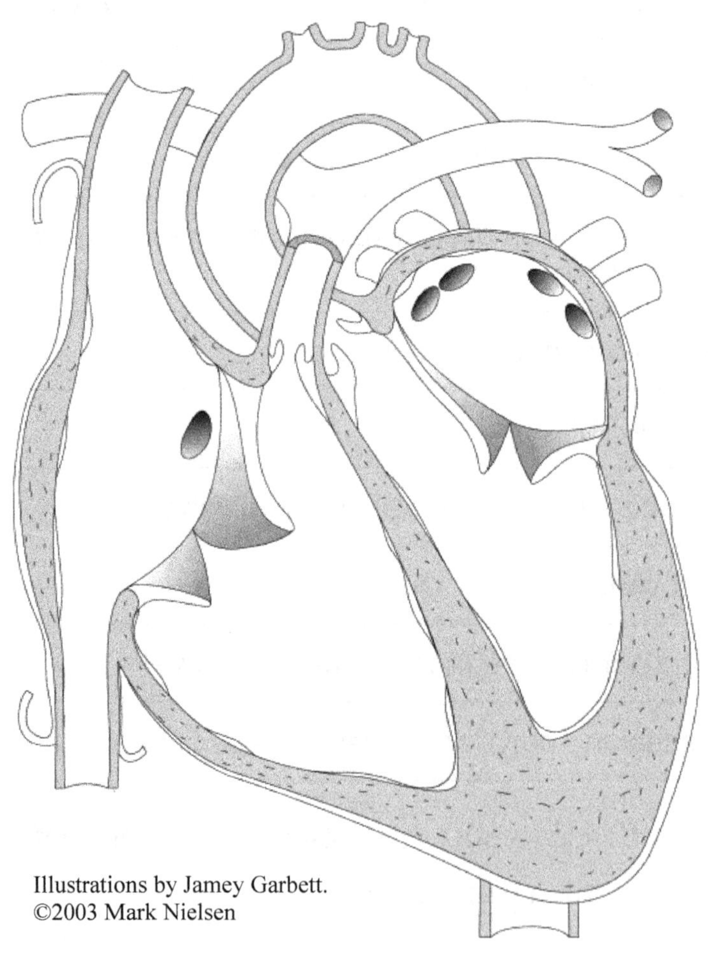

Illustrations by Jamey Garbett.
©2003 Mark Nielsen

THE FLOW OF OXYGENATED BLOOD

Once the blood leaves the left ventricle and passes through the aortic valve, it is on its way to all body tissues. The table below describes the flow of oxygenated blood to all body tissues.

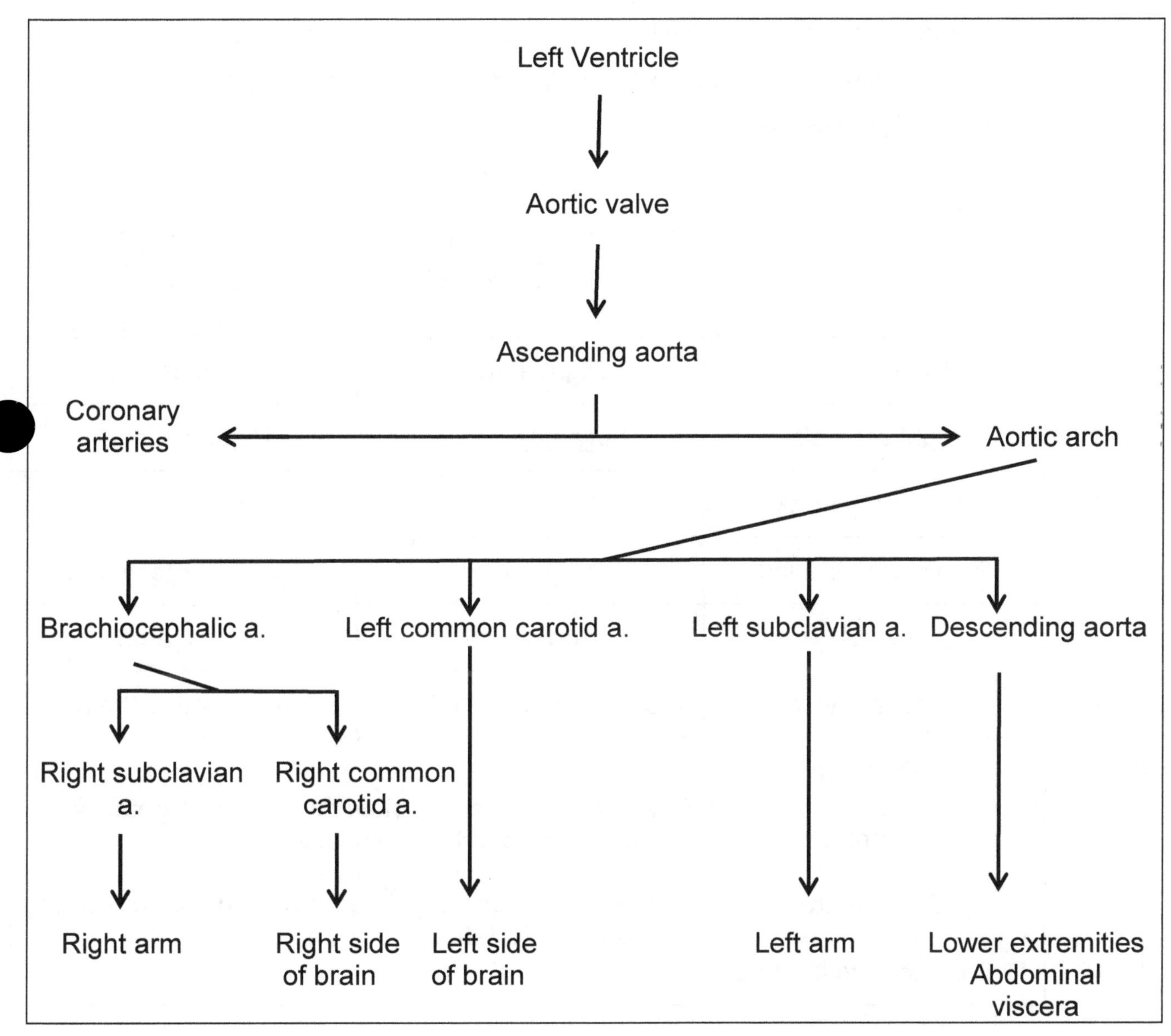

Fetal Heart

The circulation of blood through the heart of a fetus is different from the circulation of blood through an adult heart. The table below shows that the heart of a fetus has two "short cuts" or lung by passes. These short cuts are designed to get oxygenated blood to the tissues of the fetus as fast as possible. These "short cuts" are necessary because the oxygenated blood of a fetus is not fully oxygenated. As the blood of the fetus is returning from the lower extremities, it passes through the placenta to pick up oxygen (from mom) and then enters into the IVC and the right atrium. The fetal lungs are not yet functional.

steps	Adult	Fetal (Foramen Ovale) (Becomes **Fossa Ovalis** in the Adult)	Fetal (Ductus Arteriosus) (Becomes **Ligamentum Arteriosum** in the Adult)
1	Right atrium	Right atrium	Right atrium
2	Right ventricle	***Foramen ovale***	Right ventricle
3	Pulmonary trunk	Left atrium	Pulmonary trunk
4	Pulmonary arteries	Left ventricle	***Ductus arteriosus***
5	Lungs	Aortic arch	Aortic arch
6	Pulmonary veins	Deliver blood to the body	Deliver blood to the body
7	Left atrium		
8	Left ventricle	Based on this chart, it takes ten "steps" to get fully oxygenated blood to the tissues of an adult.	
9	Aortic arch	It takes six "steps" to get partially oxygenated blood to the tissues of a fetus.	
10	Deliver blood to the body		

1. Arteries transport blood away from the heart (pulmonary artery) and veins transport blood to the heart (pulmonary vein).

2. A pulmonary vessel (artery or vein) is associated with the lungs.

3. The moderator band is found only in the right ventricle.

4. The myocardium of the heart consists of cells with intercalated discs.

5. The aortic arch arches to the left and posterior to the heart.

6. The descending aorta can be subdivided to form the thoracic aorta and the abdominal aorta.

7. The bicuspid valve is actually anatomically called the "valvula bicuspidalis." However, it can be called the bicuspid valve or the mitral valve since both terms are descriptive terms.

8. The term "mitral" is in reference to the name of the hat that bishops wear. The hat is called a "mitre." Anatomists have indicated that the bicuspid valve (made of two cusps) is shaped like the hat that Bishops wear.

9. A heart murmur is a condition where one of the AV valves does not close all the way and blood from the ventricle "gurgles" back into the atrium.

10. AV valve stands for "atrioventricular valve." This would be either the tricuspid valve or the bicuspid valve.

Chapter 7C$_2$: The Torso Blood Vessels

The best way to study the blood vessels of the torso region is to start with a drop of blood in the left ventricle and follow it through the torso.

THORACIC BLOOD VESSELS

	Blood Vessels	Description
1	Left ventricle	Oxygenated blood leaves the left ventricle and passes through the aortic valve into the ascending aorta.
2	Ascending aorta	The ascending aorta leads to the aortic arch.
3	Aortic arch	The aortic arch has branches leading to the head and arms (discussed in other chapters). The aortic arch also leads to the descending aorta.
4	Descending aorta	The descending aorta extends from the arch to the hypogastric region. The portion of the descending aorta that passes through the thoracic region is called the thoracic aorta and the portion that passes through the abdomen is the abdominal aorta.
5	Thoracic aorta	The thoracic aorta branches numerous times to "feed" various thoracic organs.
6	Esophageal a	An artery that branches from the thoracic aorta to the esophagus.
7	Intercostal a	These arteries branch from the thoracic aorta to supply the rib muscles.
8	Phrenic a	These arteries branch from the thoracic aorta to supply the diaphragm muscle.

<table>
<tr><td colspan="3">Left ventricle

Ascending aorta

Aortic arch

Eventually to the subclavian arteries</td></tr>
<tr><td>1</td><td>**R. and L. Subclavian a**</td><td>The subclavian arteries lie under the clavicle and form the axillary arteries.</td></tr>
<tr><td>2</td><td>**Internal thoracic a**</td><td>These vessels branch off the subclavian arteries.

These arteries descend along the internal surface of the thorax lateral to the sternum.

These arteries supply many intercostal muscles.

These arteries also supply the mammary tissue.</td></tr>
</table>

1	**Abdominal aorta**	The abdominal aorta begins just inferior to the diaphragm muscle. It is an extension of the thoracic aorta.
2	**Celiac artery**	The celiac artery (celiac trunk) is the first branch off the abdominal aorta. Branches to form the common hepatic a. and the splenic a. The common hepatic artery supplies the liver. The splenic artery supplies the spleen. The splenic then forms the pancreatic a., and the left gastric a. The pancreatic a. supplies the pancreas. The left gastric a. supplies the stomach.
3	**Superior mesenteric a**	The superior mesenteric a. is the next branch off the abdominal aorta. Branches to supply the cecum, ascending colon, the right half of the transverse colon, and most of the small intestine. The superior mesenteric a drapes over the left renal v.
4	**Renal a**	The left and right renal arteries branch off the abdominal aorta
5	**Inferior mesenteric a**	The inferior mesenteric supplies the left half of the transverse colon, the descending colon, and the sigmoid colon.
Common Iliac a		
The descending aorta terminates at the bifurcation of the common iliac arteries, which proceed to the legs.		

After delivering oxygen to the various organs of the abdominal region, the blood eventually returns to heart. Most of the returning blood passes through the liver before arriving at the heart.

1	**Hepatic portal v**	Most of the returning blood enters the liver via the hepatic portal v.
2	**Inferior vena cava**	From the liver, the blood enters the inferior vena cava.
The inferior vena cava passes through the diaphragm muscle and enters in the right atrium of the heart.		
3	**Renal veins**	The renal veins enter directly into the inferior vena cava. Notice the left renal vein is longer than the right renal vein.

Below is some additional information regarding the blood vessels of the torso. Your instructor may add to this list.

1. Since the internal thoracic artery supplies the mammary tissue, it used to be called the internal mammary artery.

2. The hepatic portal system consists of veins entering into the liver from the abdominal viscera veins. Once inside the kidney, the blood is "cleansed" and then enters into the inferior vena cava to continue circulation.

3. Many times, if possible, the internal thoracic artery is used for coronary bypass.

4. If a patient experiences a dissected descending aorta, blood will flow rapidly into the tunica media area creating a bulge thus possibly leading to an aneurism.

Chapter 7D: The Torso Spinal Cord and Spinal Nerves

The spinal cord is part of the central nervous system and extends from the brain and passes through the magnum foramen of the skull. It is found in the posterior cavity and extends the length of the torso. Use the following tables while studying the pictures in your textbook that are associated with the spinal cord. The spinal nerves branch off the spinal cord and extend to the extremities.

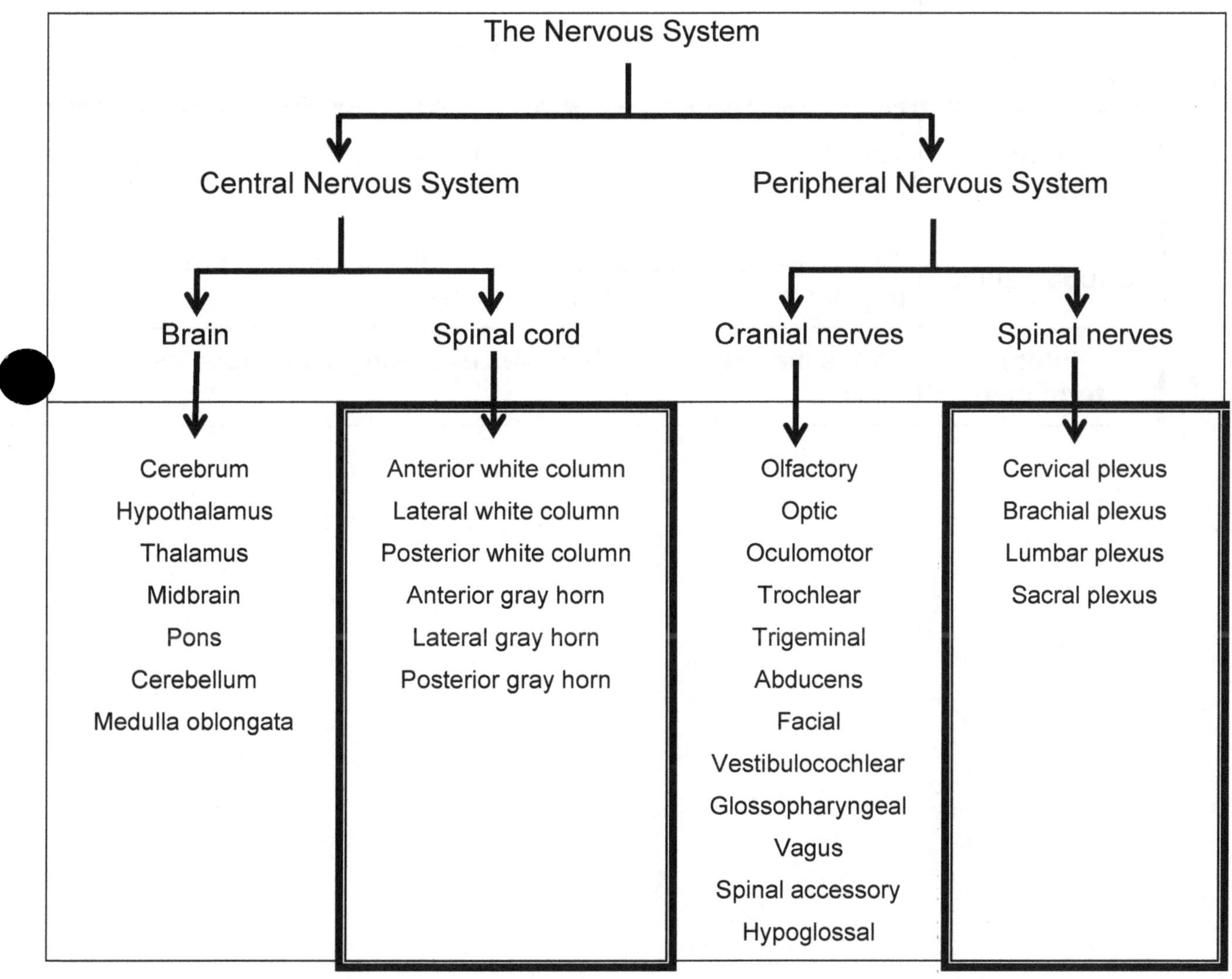

Study views of the spinal cord in your textbook while examining the table below. There are 31 pairs of nerves that emerge laterally from the spinal cord. The first pair emerges from between the skull and cervical vertebra 1 and the last nerve emerges from the coccyx region.

	Spinal Cord	Description
1	**Conus medullaris**	This is the region of the spinal cord that comes to a cone-shape in the area of lumbar-1.
2	**Cauda equina**	This is the area where the nerves of the spinal cord branch in such a manner that it looks like a horse's tail.
3	**Filum terminale**	This is the final 1, 2, or 3 nerves extending singly from the cauda equina.

While studying the table below, examine pictures of a transverse view of the spinal cord in your textbook.

	Transverse Spinal Cord	Description
1	**Anterior median sulcus**	This is a deep groove on the anterior aspect of the spinal cord. It is not as deep as the posterior median sulcus. Also call the anterior median fissure.
2	**Posterior median sulcus**	This is a deep groove on the posterior aspect of the spinal cord. It is deeper than the anterior median sulcus.
3	**Gray matter**	This is the central portion of the spinal cord. It is shaped like a butterfly or the capital letter H. The gray matter consists of: Anterior horn / Lateral horn / Posterior horn Many of the spinal nerves emerge laterally from the spinal cord by emerging from the anterior gray horn and the posterior gray horn.
4	**White matter**	This is the lighter area that surrounds the gray matter. It consists of: Anterior white / Lateral white / Posterior white The white matter consists of columns of nerves that go to and from the brain.
5	**Central canal**	This is a canal that cerebrospinal fluid flows through that is in the center of the gray matter. This is an extension of the 4th ventricle in the brain.

The table below describes select functions of the various regions of the spinal cord.

	Transverse Spinal Cord	Functions
1	**Anterior white**	This column consists of a tract of nerves (the **spinothalmic tract**) that transmits impulses (such as pain and temperature sensations) to the thalamus.
2	**Lateral white**	This column consists of a tract of nerves (the **spinocerebellar tract**) that transmits proprioception sensations to the cerebellum.
3	**Posterior white**	The posterior white consists of two major areas. One area is nearest the posterior median sulcus and the other area is lateral to it. The **fasciculus gracilis** is nearest the posterior median sulcus. The **fasciculus cuneatus** is lateral to the fasciculus gracilis. The fasciculus gracilis consists of a tract of nerves that transmits touch and pressure sensations from the lower body to the cerebrum. The fasciculus cuneatus consists of a tract of nerves that transmits touch and pressure sensations from the upper body to the cerebrum.
4	**Anterior gray**	Consists of somatic motor nerves.
5	**Lateral gray**	Consists of visceral motor nerves.
6	**Posterior gray**	Consists of somatic sensory nerves and visceral sensory nerves.

There are 31 pairs of spinal nerves that emerge laterally from the spinal cord. Examine textbook pictures while studying the table below.

	Spinal Nerves	Description
1	**Anterior rootlets**	These are branches that emerge from the anterior gray matter.
2	**Posterior rootlets**	These are branches that emerge from the posterior gray matter.
	The anterior rootlets merge together to form the anterior root. The posterior rootlets merge together to form the posterior root.	
	The anterior root and the posterior root merge together to form the spinal nerve	
	The spinal nerve branches to form the anterior ramus and the posterior ramus.	
3	**Posterior ramus**	These will branch some more to innervate back muscles (for example).
4	**Anterior ramus**	These will branch some more to innervate anterior tissues; plus, some will form nerve plexuses discussed in Chapter 5 D and 6D.

PERIPHERAL NERVES

The torso region houses the spinal cord. Branching off the spinal cord are the peripheral nerves. The peripheral nerves innervate many areas of the torso but also innervate the appendages. Some of the peripheral nerves were discussed in earlier chapters but are mentioned in this chapter as well.

The peripheral nervous system (PNS) consists of the nerves that transmit impulses from the CNS to the periphery of the body or they transmit impulses from the periphery to the CNS.   The main constituents of the PNS are the spinal nerves and the cranial nerves. The table below illustrates the various subdivisions of the peripheral nervous system (PNS). The cranial nerves are discussed in a later chapter.

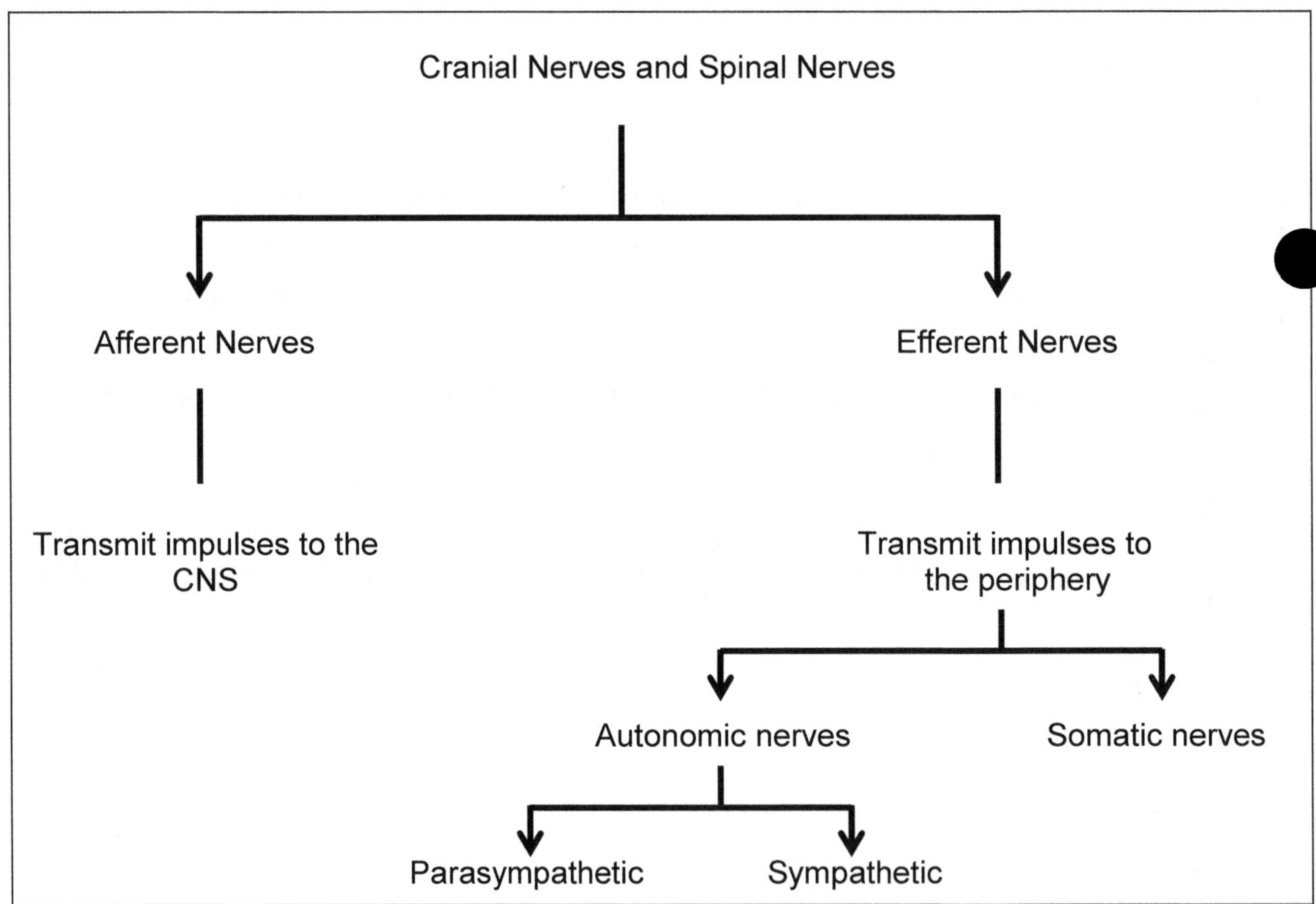

THE PLEXUSES

The table below describes the spinal nerves, specifically the plexuses that are formed. The plexuses branch to numerous areas of the body, but the table below only describes a few select nerves. Be sure to examine a picture from your textbook depicting each of the plexuses described. The plexuses were introduced in earlier chapters but are discussed in more detail in the following table.

	Plexus	Description
1	**Cervical plexus**	Consists of nerves identified as C_1 through C_8. A major nerve associated with this plexus is the phrenic nerve. This nerve innervates the diaphragm muscle.
2	**Brachial plexus**	Consists of nerves identified as C_4 through T_1. One nerve associated with this plexus is the ulnar nerve. This nerve innervates the flexor carpi ulnaris muscle.
3	**Lumbar plexus**	Consists of nerves identified as T_{12} through L_4. A major nerve associated with this plexus is the femoral nerve. This nerve innervates the sartorius and the quadriceps.
4	**Sacral plexus**	Consists of nerves identified as L_4 through S_4. A major nerve associated with this plexus is the sciatic nerve. This nerve innervates the hamstring muscles.

SYMPATHETIC AND PARASYMPATHETIC NERVES

The autonomic nerves of the peripheral nervous system (PNS) can be divided into the sympathetic division and the parasympathetic division. These divisions of the nervous system can many times be thought of as an antagonistic system (this is not always the case, however). The table below describes a few select actions comparing the sympathetic nerves with the parasympathetic nerves.

Sympathetic Action	Parasympathetic Action
The nerves from the sympathetic division emerge from the spinal cord. (T-1 through L-3)	The nerves from the parasympathetic division emerge from the brain and sacrum.
Dilates the pupil	Constricts the pupils
Increases the heart rate	Decreases the heart rate
Increases tracheal diameter	Decreases tracheal diameter
Decreases insulin production	Increases insulin production
Relaxes the urinary bladder	Tenses the urinary bladder
Causes ejaculation	Causes an erection

Conduction System		Description
1	**Sinoatrial node (SA node)**	Located on the roof of the right atrium. It is the heart's pacemaker.
2	**Atrioventricular node (AV node)**	Located on the border of the right atrium and right ventricle.
3	**Atrioventricular bundle**	This is the nerve that emerges from the AV node and then branches into the right bundle and left bundle.
4	**Right and Left bundles**	These nerves run along the interventricular septum going toward the apex of the heart.
5	**Purkinje fibers**	These nerve fibers branch off the right and left bundles and curve in such a manner as to ascend the ventricles.

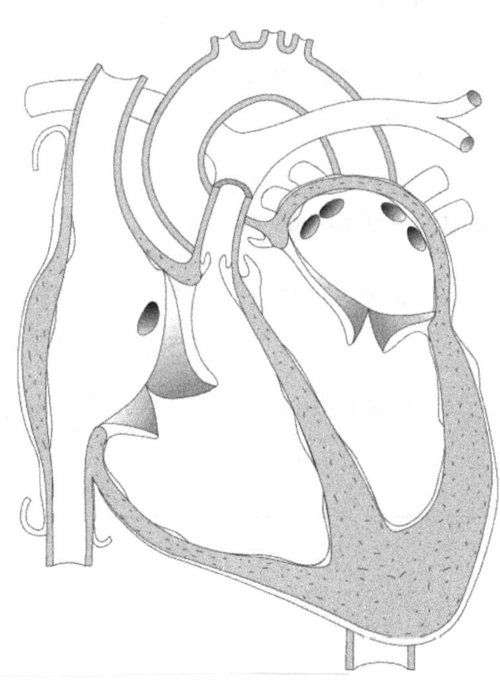

ECG (EKG)

Examine the ECG (electrocardiogram) below and then read the description that follows.

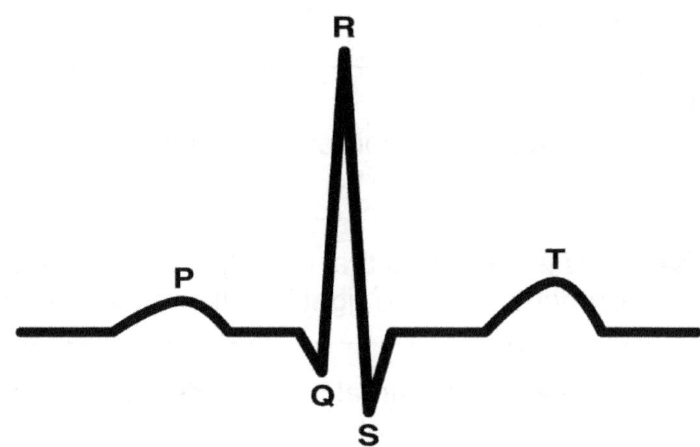

The ECG image above is labeled as P, QRS, and T waves.

P wave represents the impulses traveling from the SA node across the atria to the AV node. This is atrial contraction.

There is a flat line between the P wave and the start of the Q. This represents the impulse traveling through the AV bundles.

QRS wave represents the impulses traveling through the Purkinje fibers. This is ventricle contraction.

T wave represents ventricular repolarization. Atrial repolarization occurs during the QRS complex.

Below is some additional information regarding the nerves of the torso. Your instructor may add to this list.

1. The "bumps" associated with the ECG recording have meaning. Here are a couple of examples.

    a. If the length of the P wave is too long, this means it is taking too long for the atria to contract.
    b. If the distance between the end of the P wave and the beginning of the Q is too long, this means it is taking too long for the impulse to travel the bundle branches to cause the ventricles to contract.

2. The right and left bundle branches used to be called the Bundle of His (Hiss). Since this is a person's name, the name has been changed.

3. Purkinje is also a person's name and a suggested name change is, **subendocardial branches,** but this name really has not caught on yet.

4. ECG stands for electrocardiogram. Sometimes you will see the abbreviation EKG. This stands for electrocardiogram (British spelling).

5. The word "plexus" means "to braid."

6. Many athletic enhancement drugs are sympathetic stimulators.

Chapter 7E: The Lungs

Look at the figures in your textbook to identify the external features of the lungs.

EXTERNAL LUNG FEATURES

	Structure	Description
1	R and L lungs	The lungs are separated by the sternum in the mediastinal region.
2	Apex	This is the superior, "pointy" part of the lung.
3	Base	This is the inferior part of the lung that rests on the diaphragm muscle.
4	Lobes	Right lung: superior / middle / inferior Left lung: superior / inferior
5	Fissures	Right lung: horizontal / oblique Left lung: oblique

6	Surfaces	Each lung has the following surfaces:
		
		Diaphragmatic surface:
		        This is the surface adjacent to the diaphragm muscle.
		Mediastinal surface:
		        This is the surface adjacent to the mediastinal region.
		Costal surface:
		        This is the surface adjacent to the thoracic walls.

7	Hilum	This is the area of each lung where blood vessels enter and exit and the primary bronchi enter the lung tissue.
8	Cardiac notch	Only the left lung has the cardiac notch. Notice that the apex of the heart angles to the left and "rests" in the cardiac notch region.

The best way to study the respiratory system is to follow a molecule of air from the nasal cavity to the lungs and into the bloodstream to create oxygenated blood. Be sure to examine the figures in your textbook while studying the following tables.

Air enters through the external nares. Air becomes turbulent over the nasal conchae and any particles of debris will become stuck in the mucus lining covering the nasal conchae. Air continues to flow through the nasopharynx region.

	Structure	Description
1	**External nares**	The openings into the nasal cavity.
2	**Nasal conchae**	Three pairs of "bulges" lining the nasal cavity.
3	**Nasopharynx**	This is the general region at the posterior edge of the nasal cavity.

Air passes through the nasopharynx region and into the oropharynx region and then into the laryngopharynx region.

	Structure	Description
5	**Oropharynx**	This is the general region at the posterior edge of the mouth.
6	**Laryngopharynx**	This is the general region that is the start of the "throat."

There are several structures to discuss as air is passes through the laryngopharynx region.

	Structure	Description
1	Glottis	This is the opening to the trachea (also called the laryngeal inlet).
2	Epiglottis	This is a cartilaginous structure that causes the glottis to be either open or closed.
3	Trachea	This is the "windpipe" that is the passageway eventually leading to the lungs.

Esophagus
The esophagus is the "food tube." Notice that the esophagus is posterior to the trachea.

When food is swallowed, the food is supposed to enter into the esophagus. To ensure this, the epiglottis closes over the glottis, thereby preventing food from entering into the trachea.

Air now enters into the trachea. There are several features of the trachea to discuss.

1	Thyroid cartilage	This is the first large piece of cartilage associated with the trachea. It is wedge shaped. (Notice the location of the thyroid gland in relation to the thyroid cartilage)
2	Laryngeal prominence	This is the anterior bump of the thyroid cartilage. This bump is called the "Adam's apple" in layman's terms. Some books will call this the thyroid prominence.
3	Cricoid cartilage	This is the second cartilage on the trachea.
4	Cartilage rings	All of the other cartilage pieces on the trachea are called cartilage rings. The rings only go three-quarters of the way around the trachea.
5	Trachealis muscle	This muscle makes up the posterior portion of the trachea. It is located between the "open" ends of the three-quarter cartilage pieces.

Air leaves the trachea and enters the right and left primary bronchi at the bifurcation point called the carina.

	Structure	Description
1	**Carina**	A cartilaginous area at the distal end of the trachea that forms a "v" shaped piece of cartilage.
2	**Primary bronchi**	The right and left primary bronchi (singular = bronchus) enter into the lungs at a region called the hilum of the lung.

Notice that the right primary bronchus angles just slightly to the right and more vertical as compared to the left primary bronchus, which angles sharply to the left.

	Structure	Description
3	**Secondary bronchi**	These are the branches off the primary bronchi.
4	**Tertiary bronchi**	These are the branches off the secondary bronchi.
5	**Bronchioles**	These are the final branches of the respiratory system that terminate with alveolar sacs.
6	**Alveoli (alveolar sacs)**	These are air sacs that consist of one layer of squamous cells and are completely surrounded by blood capillaries.

The trachea and primary bronchi have cartilage rings.
The secondary and tertiary bronchi have cartilage pieces.
The bronchioles do not have any cartilage associated with them.

The function of the cartilage is support. The cartilage prevents the respiratory tubes from collapsing when a person exhales.

The secondary bronchi are smaller in diameter than the primary bronchi.
   The tertiary bronchi are smaller in diameter than the secondary bronchi.
      The bronchioles are smaller in diameter than the tertiary bronchi.

Since the bronchioles are so small in diameter, they are self-supporting. They do not require cartilage for support.

AIR ENTERING THE BLOODSTREAM

Molecules of oxygen pass through the walls of the alveolar sacs to enter into the bloodstream. Once this is accomplished, oxygen can be delivered to all body parts.

Air enters into the alveolar sacs.

Oxygen diffuses across the alveolar epithelium.

Oxygen diffuses across the capillary endothelium.

Oxygen diffuses through the red blood cell membrane.

Oxygen binds with the iron portion of the hemoglobin molecule.

The hemoglobin (within the red blood cell) transports oxygen to the left side of the heart (left atrium) via the pulmonary vein.

The oxygenated blood is ultimately pumped to all parts of the body.

In order to get air to enter the respiratory system, the thoracic cavity must enlarge. This enlargement reduces air pressure inside the thoracic cavity. Air goes from the atmosphere into the respiratory tubes.

In order to exhale, the thoracic cavity must shrink in size. This reduction in size increases air pressure inside the thoracic cavity. Air leaves the lungs and exits the body.

In order to create these pressure differences (so air can enter and exit) respiratory muscles are involved.

	Structure	Description
1	Diaphragm	This large, sheet-like muscle separates the thoracic cavity from the abdominal cavity. This muscle is innervated by the phrenic nerve, which arises from the cervical plexus. Upon contraction, this muscle extends downward, thus increasing the size of the thoracic cavity (inhalation). Upon relaxation, this muscle raises, thus decreasing the size of the thoracic cavity (exhalation).
2	Crus muscles	The right and left crus muscles help anchor the diaphragm (inferior side) to the body of the vertebrae. **Left Crus Muscle:** attached to L3. **Right Crus Muscle:** attached to L4.
3	Internal intercostal muscles	Contract in such a manner as to cause exhalation.
4	External intercostal muscles	Contract in such a manner as to cause inhalation.

THE TONSILS

The tonsils are not part of the respiratory system. They are actually part of the immune system. However, they are in the pathway of air as we inhale and exhale, so, quite often, they are discussed at this point.

	Structure	Description
1	**Pharyngeal tonsil**	Located in the nasopharynx region. Some refer to these as the adenoids. See item 3 in the "Additional Information" section.
2	**Palatine tonsils**	Located right and left lateral of the uvula in the oropharynx region.
3	**Lingual tonsil**	Located near and embedded into the base of the tongue.

Below is some additional information regarding the lungs. Your instructor may add to this list.

1. The tonsils play a minor role in our immune system.

2. Anatomically, the adenoids are called the pharyngeal tonsils.

3. Adenoid is Latin that means "like a gland." Most glands are globular in appearance; therefore, many glands are adenoids.

4. For speech to occur, the epiglottis has to be open. When swallowing food, the epiglottis has to be closed to prevent choking.

5. The trachea consists of columnar cells and goblet cells. The goblet cells produce mucus to trap inhaled debris.

6. In order to keep the alveoli from collapsing, there are special cells of the lungs (septal cells / surfactant cells / type II cells) that produce a substance called **surfactant**.

7. There are other cells of the lungs that wander around devouring possible pathogens. These are called **alveolar macrophages**.

8. The membrane surrounding the lung adjacent to it is the visceral pleura. The membrane layer that is farthest from the lung and adjacent to the thoracic wall is the parietal pleura. The space between these two layers is the pleural cavity.

9. The nasal conchae are covered by a mucus-producing membrane. This mucus traps inhaled debris; plus, the conchae themselves cause the air to become turbulent, thus warming the air before it is inhaled to the lungs.

10. The mucus membrane of the carina is the most sensitive area of the trachea and larynx for triggering a cough reflex.

11. The use of "sac" versus "sack." A sac is a physiological container or bulb that consists of gas or liquid, like "air sac." A sack is a general container that holds solid things such as groceries, tools, and sand.

Chapter 7F: The Digestive Organs

The first part of this chapter is concerned with the structures of the digestive organs. The latter part discusses briefly the digestive processes.

THE TOOTH

	Structure	Description
1	**Teeth**	Be sure to identify the teeth studied in the skull chapter. Each tooth is made of: Crown / Neck / Root.
2	**Enamel**	This is the "white" part of the tooth.
3	**Dentin**	This is the mineralized matrix that is deep to the enamel.
4	**Pulp**	This is a highly vascularized area deep to the dentin. It also consists of nerves.
5	**Periodontal ligament**	This ligament attaches the root of the tooth to the lining of the alveolar process.
6	**Apical foramen**	This is the hole at the tip of the root for the entrance and exit of blood vessels and nerves.
7	**Gingival**	This is the soft tissue in the tooth area commonly called the gum.

	Structure	Description
1	**Uvula**	This is the "hangy-down thing" in the oropharynx region.
2	**Palatoglossal arch**	This is the "arch" of tissue that extends laterally from the uvula.

3	**Tongue**	Consists of papillae
		   Which consists of taste buds
		      Which consists of gustatory cells
		         Which are associated with CN VII and send
		            signals to the brain for the interpretation of taste

4	**Lingual frenulum**	The "sliver" of tissue that anchors the tongue to the floor of the mouth
5	**Salivary glands**	There are three sets of salivary glands: **Parotid**: located near the masseter muscle **Sublingual**: located under the tongue **Submandibular**: located on the floor of the mouth.

The salivary glands produce the enzyme **salivary amylase**. This enzyme partially digests carbohydrates.

Food leaves the mouth and enters into the esophagus.

	Structure	Description
1	**Esophagus**	Located posterior to the trachea
2	**Esophageal hiatus**	The opening through the diaphragm, which the esophagus passes through

The esophagus is made of smooth muscle. The involuntary contraction of the muscle creates peristaltic waves, thus propelling food toward the stomach.

As the esophagus passes through the esophageal hiatus, it bends left and enters into the stomach.

The material passing down the esophagus is called a **bolus**.

THE STOMACH

Structure	Description
Food leaves the esophagus and enters into the stomach.	

	Structure	Description
1	Lower esophageal sphincter	This sphincter relaxes and allows food to enter the stomach.
2	Fundus	This is the large rounded portion of the stomach.
3	Pylorus	This is the distal portion of the stomach.
4	Body	The body is the region of the stomach between the fundus area and the pylorus area.
5	Pyloric sphincter	This sphincter is in the pylorus area and, when it relaxes, food passes into the duodenum of the small intestine.
6	Lesser curvature	This is the small curve of the stomach located along the superior edge.
7	Greater curvature	This is the large curve of the stomach located along the inferior edge.

	Structure	Description
8	**Lesser omentum**	Peritoneal tissue that attaches to the lesser curvature of the stomach and the liver.
9	**Greater omentum**	Peritoneal tissue that attaches to the greater curvature of the stomach and extends over the small intestine to the distal aspect of the abdomen.
10	**Gastric rugae**	These are muscular folds that make up the inside lining of the stomach, which allows it to stretch when food enters. A stomach consisting of lots of rugae has had very little food in it recently. A stomach consisting of very few rugae has recently had food in it.
11	**Stomach musculature**	There are three major sets of muscles associated with the stomach: **Circular muscles**: When these muscles contract, the stomach "squeezes" inward. **Longitudinal muscles**: When these muscles contract, the stomach "squeezes" superior to inferior. **Oblique muscles**: When these muscles contract, the stomach twists.

The stomach produces the enzyme **pepsin**. Pepsin partially digests protein.

The partially digested material is now called acidic **chyme**.

THE SMALL INTESTINE

Food leaves the stomach and enters into the small intestine.

	Structure	Description
1	**Duodenum**	The first part of the small intestine. It is approximately 1 foot in length. Most of the chemical digestion occurs here.
2	**Jejunum**	The second part of the small intestine. It is approximately 8 feet in length. Most of the nutrients are absorbed into the bloodstream from the jejunum.
3	**Ileum**	The third part of the small intestine. It is approximately 10 to 12 feet in length. This part connects to the cecum (the first part of the large intestine). Some nutrient absorption occurs here, but absorption of vitamins is the main function of the ileum.

The major function of the small intestine is to digest food and absorb nutrients into the bloodstream.

	Structure	Description
4	**Villi**	Villi line the inside border of the small intestine. Nutrients are absorbed through the villi to enter into capillaries and then be transported to all body tissues.

The small intestine produces the following select digestive enzymes:

Maltase / **Sucrase** / **Lactase**: These enzymes digest carbohydrates.

Peptidase: This enzyme digests protein.

THE LARGE INTESTINE

	Material leaves the small intestine and enters into the large intestine.	
	Structure	**Description**
1	**Cecum**	The first part of the large intestine. The appendix also attaches to the cecum.
2	**Ascending colon**	Fecal matter is transported "up" the ascending colon, which is on the right side of the abdomen.
3	**Hepatic flexure**	This is the bend of the large intestine leading to the transverse colon (near the liver).
4	**Transverse colon**	Fecal matter is transported to the left side of the body.
5	**Splenic flexure**	This is the bend of the large intestine leading to the descending colon (near the spleen).
6	**Descending colon**	Fecal matter is transported "down" the descending colon, which is on the left side of the abdomen.
7	**Sigmoid flexure**	This is the bend of the large intestine leading to the sigmoid colon.
8	**Sigmoid colon**	This is the last segment of the large intestine. Fecal matter is transported through the sigmoid colon leading to the rectum.
9	**Rectum**	This is an expandable organ for temporary storage of fecal matter.
10	**Anus**	The entrance to the anus consists of the internal anal sphincter (involuntary control). The exit of the anus consists of the external anal sphincter (voluntary control).

Structure		Description
11	**Taeniae coli**	This is the longitudinal, smooth muscle of the large intestine.
12	**Haustra**	These are the circular, smooth muscles of the large intestine.
13	**Ileocecal valve**	(Ileocecal sphincter) This is the sphincter located at the entrance to the cecum from the ileum.

There are two major muscles involved with the large intestine.

The **appendix** is not a part of the digestive system, but it is attached to the cecum of the large intestine.

Most textbooks will draw the appendix in the **"pelvic position"** (hanging in a downward position from the cecum). However, 65% of appendices are in a **"retrocecal" position** (laying on the cecum, parallel to the taeniae coli).

THE LARGE INTESTINE SELECT FUNCTIONS

The large intestine does more than simply get rid of solid waste.

1	Gets rid of solid waste
2	Prevents dehydration
3	Houses bacteria that produce vitamin K, which is used for some blood clotting factors.

The Small and Large Intestine

Small Intestine	Large Intestine
About 20 feet in length duodenum = 1 ft. jejunum = 8 ft. ilium = 10 to12 ft.	About 5 feet in length
About 2 inches in diameter	About 3.5 inches in diameter
Digests and absorbs nutrients	Does not digest but it will absorb water
Uses peristalsis to push material (chyme) through	Uses peristalsis to push fecal matter through

THE LIVER

The liver, pancreas, and gallbladder are considered to be accessory structures of digestion. These organs produce, secrete, or produce and secrete products into the small intestine that are used in the digestive processes. Food does not enter into them to be digested.

The following are features you can see from an anterior view of the liver.

	Structure	Description
1	**Lobes**	There is a rather large left lobe and a small right lobe of the liver.
2	**Falciform ligament**	This is the ligament found between the right and left lobes of the liver. It attaches the liver to the anterior abdominal wall.
3	**Coronary ligament**	This is the ligament that "branches" off the falciform ligament and "runs" along the superior edge of the liver, thus attaching to the inferior side of the diaphragm muscle.
4	**Round ligament**	This ligament is an extension of the falciform ligament. It connects to the umbilicus. This ligament is the remnant of the umbilical vessels.
5	**Gallbladder**	From an anterior view, the gallbladder appears to be a small organ. Lift the liver up to see the rest of the gallbladder. It is larger than it appears. The gallbladder stores bile.

Bile is not an enzyme and does not digest anything. Bile emulsifies fat that is in the small intestine. This makes it easier for the enzymes to digest the fat.

THE LIVER AND GALLBLADDER

The following are structures involved with the flow of bile from the liver to the duodenum, from the gallbladder to the duodenum, and also the flow of bile that fills the gallbladder.

FLOW OF BILE

Flow of Bile from Liver to Duodenum	Flow of Bile from Gallbladder to Duodenum	Flow of Bile from Liver to Gallbladder
Hepatocytes	Cystic duct	Hepatocytes
R and L hepatic ducts	Common bile duct	R and L hepatic ducts
Common hepatic duct	Hepatopancreatic sphincter	Common hepatic duct
Common bile duct	Sphincter is open	Common bile duct
Hepatopancreatic sphincter	Duodenum	Hepatopancreatic sphincter
Sphincter is open		Sphincter is closed
Duodenum		Common bile duct
		Cystic duct
		Gallbladder

THE PANCREAS

The pancreas is heavily involved in the digestive process. The pancreas produces numerous enzymes, which leave the pancreas, pass through the hepatopancreatic sphincter, and enter into the duodenum of the small intestine. It is in the small intestine that the pancreatic enzymes digest food.

The following are features of the pancreas		
	Structure	**Description**
1	**Head**	This is the part of the pancreas that is adjacent to the duodenum of the small intestine.
2	**Body**	This is the main portion of the pancreas.
3	**Tail**	This is the small "pointy" end of the pancreas. It is the area that is nearest the spleen.
4	**Pancreatic lobules**	The surface of the pancreas consists of nodules called pancreatic lobules. These lobules consist of two types of cells: **Acinar cells**: produce digestive enzymes **Pancreatic islet cells**: produce hormones

SELECT FUNCTIONS OF THE PANCREAS

The table below describes the functions of the pancreas. The pancreas consists of many lobules. Lobules consist of acinar cells and pancreatic islet cells.

	Structure	Select Function
1	**Acinar cells produce: (enzymes)**	**Carbohydrases**: digest carbohydrates (<u>amylase</u>) **Proteinases**: digest protein (<u>trypsin</u>, <u>chymotrypsin</u>, <u>carboxypeptidase</u>) **Lipases**: digest lipids (<u>lipase</u>)
2	**Pancreatic islet cells produce: (hormones)**	**Insulin**: Opens protein channels in the cell membrane, thus allowing glucose to leave the bloodstream and enter into the cell. **Glucagon**: Causes the liver to begin to break down the stored glycogen, thus putting glucose into the bloodstream. **Somatostatin**: Regulates the release of growth hormone from the pituitary gland—helps regulate growth.

Flow of digestive enzymes into the duodenum:

Enzymes leave the acinar cells.
Enter into the pancreatic duct.
Travel to the hepatopancreatic sphincter.
Enter into the duodenum of the small intestine.

Below is some additional information regarding the digestive organs. Your instructor may add to this list.

1. The stomach does very little digestion.

2. The small intestine does the majority of the digestion.

3. The small intestine produces numerous enzymes, plus it also gets a host of enzymes from the pancreas to digest food.

4. Bile does not digest food. Bile emulsifies fat to make it easier for lipase to digest the fat.

5. The hepatic flexure is also called the right colic flexure and the splenic flexure is also called the left colic flexure.

6. Ulcers result from the breakdown of the lining of either the stomach (stomach ulcer) or the duodenum (duodenal ulcer). Researchers now believe that the majority of ulcers are due to a bacterium (***Helicobacter pylori***).

7. Rapid peristalsis of the large intestine results in diarrhea and slow peristalsis results in constipation.

8. The tail of the pancreas is positioned to the left side of the body.

9. Most of the stomach is on the left side of the midline of the body.

10. The greater omentum has an attachment at the greater curvature of the stomach but no attachment at the lower end of the abdomen.

11. The term "jejunum" comes from Latin that means "fasting." When early anatomists cut into a dead patient's small intestine, they found this portion to be devoid of food.

12. The enzymes that digest carbohydrates are collectively call carbohydrases.

13. The enzymes that digest protein are collectively called proteinases.

14. The enzymes that digest lipids are collectively called lipases.

Chapter 8:   The Pelvic Region

The pelvic region is inferior to the abdomen and superior to the legs. The study of the pelvic region is designed differently from the study of the other body regions. The study of the pelvic region is divided in the following manner:

8.A.   This chapter discusses the urinary system. In this class, we will study the structure of the kidney and the nephrons in detail. Then we study the blood vessels associated with the internal kidney. There is a discussion relating to the following:

    a. Flow of blood to and from the kidney.

    b. Flow of water to and from the kidney.

    c. Flow of waste products to the kidney and out of the body.

8.B.   This chapter discusses the male reproductive system. In this class, we will study the structures of the male reproductive system, which includes the following:

    a. Passage of sperm from the testes to ejaculation.

    b. The attachment of the penis to the pelvic region.

8.C.   This chapter discusses the female reproductive system. In this class, we will study the structures of the female reproductive system, which includes the following:

    a. Passage of a fertilized egg to the implantation in the endometrium.

    b. Passage of sperm through the female system to the fertilization of the egg.

    c. Anchoring the uterus to the pelvic region.

Chapter 8A: The Urinary System

As the body utilizes the nutrients obtained from the digestion of food, waste products are produced. Some of these waste products exit the body in the form of feces in the large intestine, while other wastes leave the body via the urinary system. View images from your textbook as you study the following tables.

The Gross Anatomy of the Urinary System

Follow a particle of waste through the urinary system beginning in the descending aorta.	
Structure	**Description**
1 **Renal artery**	Material enters into the left and right kidney from the left and right renal arteries. (Note: the right renal artery goes "under" the inferior vena cava.)
2 **Kidneys**	The kidneys are retroperitoneal. The left kidney is positioned in the body just a bit higher than the right kidney, due to the size of the liver. Waste is processed within the tubules inside the kidneys.
3 **Ureters**	The ureters exit the kidneys at the area of the hilum. The ureters enter the urinary bladder.
4 **Urinary bladder**	Urine begins to fill the urinary bladder and eventually the urinary bladder contracts to void the urine. The urinary bladder is in the pelvic region of the body.
5 **Urethra**	Urine leaves the urinary bladder to pass through the urethra.
After the arteries transport waste to the kidneys, the waste is processed and enters ihto tubules inside the kidneys. Then, the "cleaned" blood returns to circulation in the following manner:	
6 **Renal veins**	The right and left renal veins enter the inferior vena cava. (Note: the left renal vein is longer than the right and has to go "over" the surface of the descending aorta).
7 **Inferior vena cava**	The inferior vena cava passes through the diaphragm muscle and eventually enters into the right atrium of the heart.

This table describes the overall structure of the kidneys. The next table describes the details of the nephrons of the kidney. Be sure to look at an image of the sagittal view of the kidney while studying the following tables.

	Structure	Description
1	Renal cortex	These are the three main regions of the kidney. Many nephrons (kidney tubules) are located in the renal cortex.
2	Renal medulla	
3	Renal pelvis	
4	Renal pyramids	There are usually six to eighteen renal pyramids located within the renal medulla area.
5	Renal columns	This is the space between each of the renal pyramids.

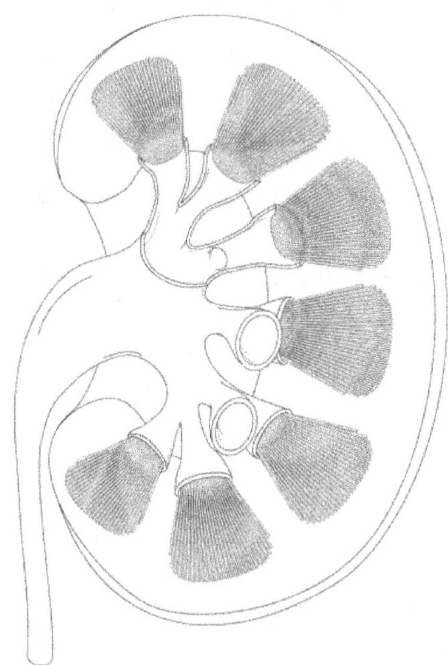

Illustrations by Jamey Garbett.
©2003 Mark Nielsen

NEPHRONS

This table describes the nephrons of the kidneys. The next table describes the details of the circulatory pattern of the kidney. Be sure to look at an image of the sagittal view of the kidney while studying the following tables.

Now, imagine this: the waste products the kidney is disposing of begin in the nephrons located in the renal cortex. Follow a waste particle from the renal cortex to the ureter.		
	Structure	**Description**
1	**Nephron**	These are the main functioning units of the kidney that are involved in processing the waste. **Glomerular capsule**: This is the first part of the nephron. **Proximal convoluted tubule (PCT)**: This is the second part of the nephron. It is a highly coiled tubule. **Nephron loop:** This is the third part of the nephron. This loop extends into the renal medulla area. **Distal convoluted tubule (DCT)**: This is the fourth part of the nephron. It is also a highly coiled tubule.
2	**Collecting tubule**	Waste leaves the DCT of the various nephrons and enters (collects) into the collecting tubules. These tubules appear as "stripes" in the renal pyramids.
3	**Minor calyx**	Waste in the collecting tubules merges together to collect in the minor calyx, which is located at the distal end of each renal pyramid.
4	**Major calyx**	Waste in each minor calyx merges together to collect in a major calyx.
5	**Renal pelvis**	Waste in each major calyx merges together to collect in the renal pelvis region.
6	**Ureter**	Waste from the renal pelvis enters into the ureter.

BLOOD VESSELS OF THE KIDNEY

This table describes the circulatory system of the kidneys. Be sure to look at an image of the sagittal view of the kidney while studying the following tables.

	Structure	Description
	Begin with a particle of waste in the renal artery and follow it through kidneys.	
1	**Renal artery**	The renal artery enters the hilum area of the kidney.
2	**Segmental a.**	This artery branches off the renal artery. There are usually two or three segmental arteries.
3	**Interlobar a.**	These arteries pass through the renal column area on their way to the renal cortex area.
4	**Arcuate a.**	This artery "runs" along the border of the renal cortex and renal medulla.
5	**Interlobular a.**	Also called the **radiate artery**. This artery extends into the renal cortex, on its way to the glomerular capsule area.
6	**Afferent arteriole**	The afferent arteriole enters into the glomerular capsule area.
7	**Glomerular capillaries**	Once material enters the glomerular capillaries, it can be forced (due to blood pressure) into the capsular area and then into the PCT.
8	**Efferent arteriole**	The efferent arteriole leaves the glomerular capillaries and exits the glomerular region. It will then lead to the peritubular capillaries.
9	**Peritubular capillaries**	These capillaries surround portions of the PCT and the DCT. As soon as the capillaries straighten out and run parallel to the nephron loop area, they are called the vasa recta.
10	**Vasa recta**	These vessels run parallel to the nephron loop. The term "recta" means straight.

This is a sagittal view of the kidney to show the blood vessels that are involved with transporting waste to the nephrons of the kidney.

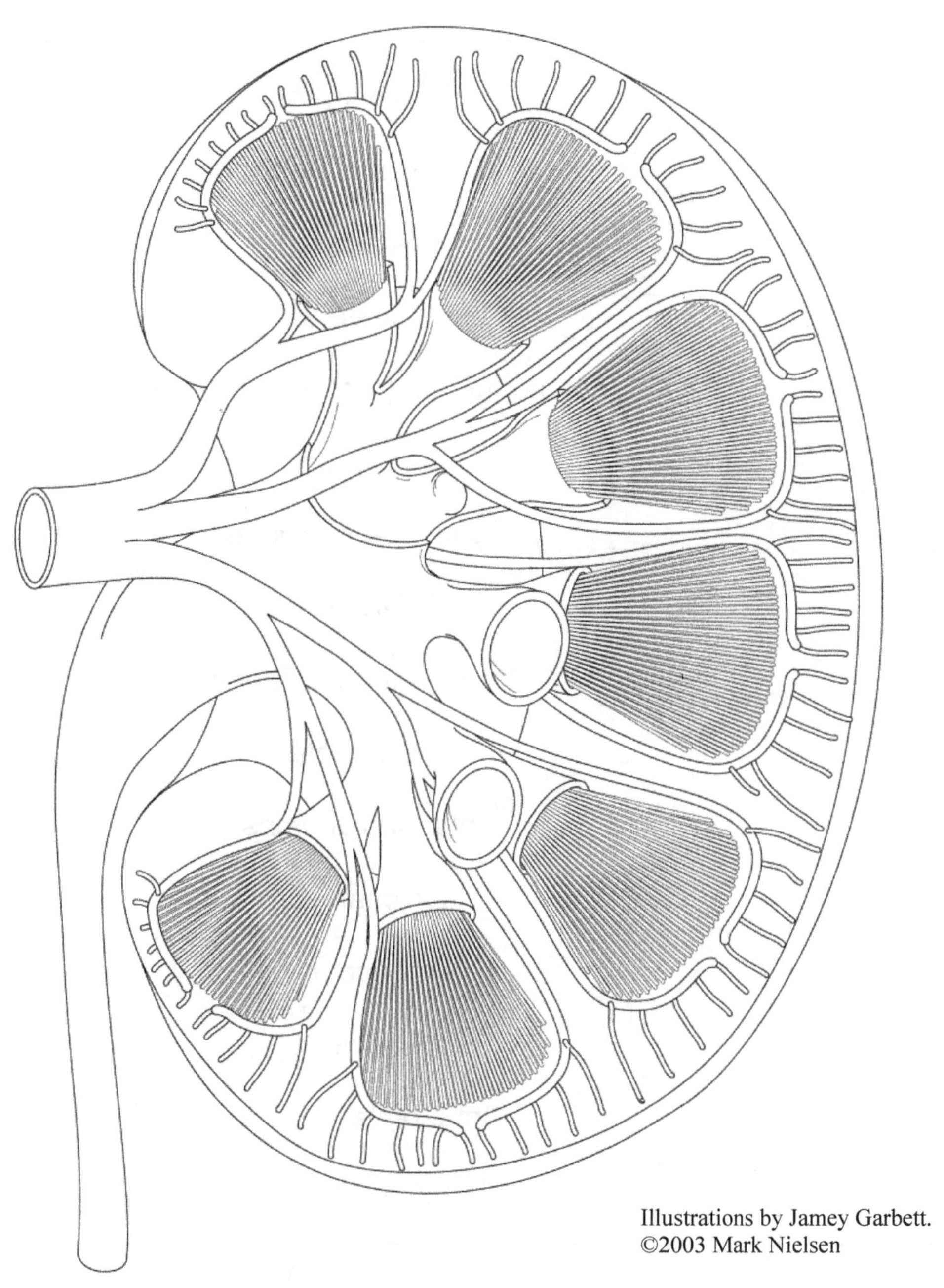

Illustrations by Jamey Garbett.
©2003 Mark Nielsen

The blood that leaves the vasa recta will enter into a series of veins that parallel the arteries discussed in the previous table. The table below lists the flow of blood from the renal artery to the right atrium of the heart. Notice, there is not a segmental vein.

Renal artery
Segmental artery
Interlobar a.
Arcuate a.
Interlobular a. (cortical radiate a.)
Afferent a.
Glomerular capillaries
Efferent a.
Peritubular capillaries
Vasa recta
Interlobular veins
Arcuate v
Interlobar v
Renal v
Inferior vena cava
Right atrium of the heart

WATER / WASTE / BLOOD

This table describes more detailed functions of the nephrons. Blood transports material to the nephron, and it consists of: waste products, erythrocytes, and water. The table below describes the flow of each of these entities regarding how the nephrons function.

The Flow of Waste	The Flow of Water		The Flow of Blood
Renal a	Renal a		Renal a
Segmental a	Segmental a		Segmental a
Interlobar a	Interlobar a		Interlobar a
Arcuate a	Arcuate a		Arcuate a
Cortical radiate a	Cortical radiate a		Cortical radiate a
Afferent a	Afferent a		Afferent a
Glomerular capillaries	Glomerular capillaries		Glomerular capillaries
Nephron	Nephron	Efferent a	Efferent a
Toilet		Peritubular capillaries	Peritubular capillaries
		Cortical radiate v	Cortical radiate v
		Arcuate v	Arcuate v
		Interlobar v	Interlobar v
		Renal v	Renal v

URINARY BLADDER AND URETHRA

This table describes the urinary bladder structures.

	Structure	Description
1	**Ureteral openings**	The ureters enter the urinary bladder on the posterior-inferior portion of the urinary bladder.
2	**Vesicoureteral sphincters**	This is the muscular portion around the ureteral openings. It is not a true sphincter or a true valve.
3	**Trigone**	This is the smooth triangular area that is between the ureteral openings and the urethral opening.
4	**Urethra**	This is the urinary tube that exits the urinary bladder.
5	**Internal urethral sphincter**	This sphincter is involuntary and is located at the exit of the urinary bladder. In males, it is located superior to the prostate gland.
6	**External urethral sphincter**	This sphincter is voluntary and is located about 3 cm inferior to the internal urethral sphincter. In males, it is located at the inferior edge of the prostate gland.
7	**Detrusor muscle**	This muscle makes up the urinary bladder wall.

1. Cortical nephrons are located mainly in the cortex region of the kidney.

2. Juxtamedullary nephrons have longer nephron loops and are located mainly in the medulla region of the kidney. The glomerular capsule region usually is on the border of the renal cortex and renal medulla.

3. The glomerular capsule and glomerular capillaries are the site for the filtering apparatus of the kidneys.

4. Of the kidney's nephrons, 85% are cortical nephrons and 15% are juxtamedullary nephrons.

5. "Juxta" is Latin that means "close to." For example, the juxtamedullary nephrons are close to the medulla region of the kidneys.

6. The striped appearance of the renal pyramids is due to the numerous collecting tubules associated with the nephrons.

7. The juxtaglomerular cells are located on the afferent and efferent arterioles in the region of the vascular pole of the glomerular capsule.

8. There are numerous nephrons that "connect" to the collecting tubule. All nephrons connect to the collecting tubule via the distal convoluted tubule.

9. An afferent arteriole enters the glomerular capsule and an efferent arteriole exits the glomerular capsule.

10. It looks like waste products have to travel through several parts of the nephron before exiting the body. The reason: each part of the nephron has specific functions regarding either adding material to the urine or removing material from the urine. This is called "processing the urine." This is learned in more detail in a physiology course.

11. Upon contraction of the urinary bladder to void, the tissue around the ureteral openings "pinches" shut, thereby preventing urine from back-flowing into the ureters.

12. Since the tissue in the area of the ureteral openings "pinches closed," it is not a true valve or sphincter.

13. The urinary bladder will stretch to accommodate a little more than 800 mL of urine.

14. At approximately 200 mL, the urinary bladder stretches enough to send signals to the brain to begin the urge to void.

15. At approximately 400 mL, the internal urethral sphincter opens involuntarily.

16. At approximately 800 mL, the external urethral sphincter opens due to the pressure. This sphincter is under voluntary control but, with enough pressure, it will open automatically.

17. The combination of the glomerular capsule and the glomerular capillaries is called the glomerulus.

18. The trigone area acts as a funnel to direct urine toward the urethra. Also, when the trigone stretches, a signal is sent to the brain indicating it is time to think about going to the bathroom.

Chapter 8B: The Reproductive System (Male)

Look at the figures in your textbook to identify the structures of the male reproductive system.

The Male Reproductive System

	Structure	Description
	Follow the path of sperm as it travels through the male reproductive system.	
1	**Seminiferous tubules**	These tubes are inside the testes. The cells lining these tubes produce sperm cells. Sperm cells are produced due to the action of the follicle stimulating hormone from the pituitary gland.
2	**Efferent ductules**	These tubes extend from the seminiferous tubules to the epididymis.
3	**Epididymis**	This is a highly coiled structure on the posterior-outer edge of the testes.
4	**Ductus deferens**	The epididymis uncoils and forms a singular tube (vas deferens).
	The ductus deferens extends upward from the epididymis, loops around the urinary bladder, and descends back toward the penile urethra of the penis.	
5	**Ejaculatory duct**	This tube extends from the ductus deferens into the prostate gland and merges with the prostatic urethra (from the urinary bladder) to form the penile urethra.
6	**Penile urethra**	This urethra extends from the prostatic urethra to the external urethral orifice of the penis. It is sometimes called the spongy urethra.

Look at the figures in your textbook to identify the layers of the scrotum.

Structures of the Scrotum

Begin with the outermost layer of the scrotum and remove tissue layer by layer.

	Structure	Description
1	**Skin**	The outermost layer of the scrotal sac
2	**Dartos muscle**	Deep to the skin layer. These smooth muscles give the scrotal skin its characteristic wrinkling.
3	**Superficial scrotal fascia**	Also called the dartos fascia. This layer is deep to the dartos muscles.
4	**Cremaster muscle**	These are longitudinal, skeletal muscles that surround the testes (connecting to the tunica vaginalis layer) and extend upward into the spermatic cord, eventually merging with the internal oblique muscle.
5	**Tunica vaginalis**	This is a double-layered pouch that surrounds the testes. **Parietal layer**: this is the outermost layer of the tunica vaginalis. **Visceral layer**: this is the innermost layer of the tunica vaginalis. There is a cavity between the parietal and visceral layers.
6	**Tunica albuginea**	This layer is deep to the tunica vaginalis and is on the surface of the testes. This is considered to be the outer layer of the testes.

TESTES

Look at the figures in your textbook to identify the structures of the testes.

Structures of the Testes

	Structure	Description
1	**Seminiferous tubules**	These are highly coiled tubes inside the testes. Sperm production occurs inside these tubules. Each tubule is about 30 inches in length.
2	**Lobules**	The seminiferous tubules are arranged in roughly 800 sections called lobules
3	**Septa**	Each lobule is divided by a septa. Each septa is lined with an extension of the tunica albuginea.
4	**Mediastinum of the testes**	All of the lobules converge to one area of the testes called the mediastinum.
5	**Rete testis**	All the seminiferous tubules form a smaller coil of tubules called the rete testis, which is located in the mediastinum.
6	**Efferent ductules**	These ducts lead from the rete testis to the head of the epididymis.
7	**Epididymis**	The head of the epididymis consists of coiled tubules, and as the tubules extend to the tail of the epididymis, they become less coiled to eventually form a single tube exiting the epididymis (ductus deferens).
8	**Ductus deferens**	The single tube exiting the epididymis and leading toward the penile urethra

The table below discusses some additional information regarding the testes.

Additional Information
Cremaster muscle: Normal sperm development in the seminiferous tubules requires a temperature around 96.6° F. The rest of the body functions at a temperature of 98.6°F. Therefore, the testes are on the outside of the body in order to maintain a temperature approximately 2° cooler than the rest of the body. When the outside temperature drops too low, the cremaster muscles contract to "pull" the testes closer to the abdomen in order to maintain the correct temperature for sperm development.
Ductus deferens: Prior to birth, the testicle development occurs inside the abdominal cavity of the fetus at about the location of the kidneys. Therefore, the vas deferens extends from the "higher-positioned" testes straight down toward the penile urethra. As fetal development continues, the testes descend, and the ductus deferens forms a loop around the ureters. Then, the testes descend all the way to the scrotal sac on the outside of the body. As a result of this testicle migration, the sperm now leave the testes and travel "up" the ductus deferens, "around" the ureters, and then "back down" toward the penile urethra.

● ACCESSORY GLANDS

There are three glands that provide various products for sperm survival.

	Structure	Description
1	**Seminal gland (2 glands)**	Also called the **seminal vesicle gland**. These glands are located posterior to the urinary bladder and close to the superior surface of the prostate gland. The contents of the seminal gland enter into the ejaculatory duct. These glands provide about 60% of the volume of semen. This semen consists of a high concentration of fructose, which provides nutrients for the sperm cells as they travel through the reproductive system on their way to find an egg to fertilize.
2	**Prostate gland (1 gland)**	This gland is located inferior to the urinary bladder and anterior to the rectum. This gland is normally about 4 cm in diameter. This gland provides about 20–30% of the volume of semen. This semen is slightly acidic and has been found to consist of seminal plasmin, which is an antibiotic, which probably helps prevent urinary tract infections. This semen enters directly into the prostatic urethra.
3	**Bulbo-urethral gland (2 glands)**	These glands are located at the base of the penis, slightly inferior to the prostate gland. These are small bulbs with a diameter of about 10 mm. This semen is alkaline, which helps to neutralize the acid nature of urine that might be present in the urethra. This semen is also a fairly thick mucus material that provides lubrication for the tip of the penis. This semen enters directly into the penile urethra.

PENIS

Look at the figures in your textbook to identify the structures of the penis. The best view to use is a sagittal view.

Structures of the Penis

	Structure	Description
1	Shaft of the penis	This is the main body of the penis. Inside the shaft of the penis are erectile tissues (discussed later).
2	Glans	This is the tissue at the distal end of the penis.
3	External urethral orifice	This is the central opening at the distal end of the glans.
4	Corpus cavernosum	There are two cylindrical erectile tissues located on the anterior side of a flaccid penis or what appears to be on the superior surface of an erect penis. These erectile tissues have an artery (deep artery of the penis) in the center. Between the two corpora cavernosa is a vein (deep dorsal vein of the penis). Blood flows into the penis via the two deep arteries and returns to the body via the single deep vein. This flow of blood in and out of the penis is involved in the development of an erection (discussed later).
5	Corpus spongiosum	This tissue is deep to the two corpora cavernosa. This tissue encircles the penile urethra.
6	Bulb of the penis	This is an expanded area of the corpus spongiosum at the proximal end of the penis near the prostate gland.

PENIS ATTACHMENT

Look at the figures in your textbook to identify the structures that are involved in attaching the penis to the body.

Attachment of the Penis to the Pelvis

	Structure	Description
1	Crus of the penis	There are a right crus and a left crus. The crura (plural of crus) are extensions of the corpora cavernosa. The right and left crura attach to the ischial ramus (the region between the ischium and the pubis of the pelvic bone).
2	Bulb of the penis	The bulb is surrounded by the bulbospongiosus muscle.
3	Bulbospongiosus muscle	This muscle merges with the superficial transverse perineal muscle and the crus of the penis.
4	Superficial transverse perineal muscle	This muscle extends from the left ischial ramus to the right ischial ramus and joins together in the middle at the perineal body
5	Perineal body	This area expands to form a muscle that merges with the external anal sphincter muscle.
6	External anal sphincter muscle	This muscle encircles the anus and the posterior portion attaches to the coccyx.
7	Suspensory ligament of the penis	This ligament extends from the crus of the penis to the pubic symphysis.
8	Ischiocavernosus muscle	This muscle covers the crus of the penis and attaches to the ramus of the ischium.

THE REPRODUCTIVE SYSTEM (MALE):
ADDITIONAL INFORMATION

1. Vas deferens is Latin for "vessel that carries away." Vas is "vessel" and deferens is "carry away." This is also called the ductus deferens. Ductus refers to a tube.

2. Most (if not all) male mammals have descended testes.

3. The testes have to descend out of the abdominal cavity in order to have a temperature about 2° cooler than the body. Sperm cells cannot develop at 98.6°.

4. An erection is due to stimulation of the sympathetic nerves that cause the penile artery to dilate. Therefore, more blood rushes into the penis; but, since the vein that exits the penis does not dilate, the result is a "backlog" of blood in the penis.

5. Ejaculation is due to the activation of different nerves that result in peristaltic activity of the vas deferens and the seminal gland.

6. A vasectomy is performed by making an incision on the posterior side of the scrotal sac and cutting the vas deferens. Sperm can still be produced but cannot travel through the vas deferens.

7. Epididymis is Latin for "on the testes." "Epi" is reference to "on" and "didymos" is in reference to "testes."

8. Cremaster is Latin for "to suspend."

9. Vas deferens and ductus deferens refer to the same tube.

10. The testes normally descend by the age of 9 months. If they do not descend, the child needs to be evaluated because undescended testes could result in sterility.

Chapter 8C: The Reproductive System (Female)

Look at the figures in your textbook to identify the structures of the female reproductive system. Begin the study of the female reproductive system with the uterus.

The Female Reproductive System

	Structure	Description
1	**Uterus**	This is a pear-shaped organ that is about 7 cm long and 5 cm in width at its widest part.
2	**Fundus of uterus**	This is the superior, rounded portion of the uterus.
3	**Lining of the uterus**	**Endometrial lining**: This is the innermost lining. During pregnancy and ovulation it will become thicker to allow for implantation of a fertilized egg. **Myometrium**: This is the thick muscular portion that is involved in uterine contractions during labor. **Perimetrium**: This is the outermost layer of the uterus.
4	**Cervix**	This is the apical end of the uterus.
5	**External os of uterus**	This is the opening into the uterus at the apical end surrounded by the cervix tissue.
6	**Uterine tube**	These tubes extend laterally from the fundus of the uterus toward the ovaries.
7	**Fimbriae**	These are finger-like projections from the uterine tubes that come in close contact with the ovaries.
8	**Ovaries**	These are paired organs located near the walls of the pelvic cavity. Each ovary is about 5 cm long and 2.5 cm wide.

FERTILIZED EGG

Look at the figures in your textbook to identify the structures of the female reproductive system while following a sperm cell to the site of fertilization of the egg and to the implantation of a fertilized egg.

Fertilization and Implantation of an Egg

	Structure	Description
1	Vagina	This is an elastic muscular tube (7.5-9 cm long) that extends from the external genitalia of the female to the cervix of the uterus.

Ovulation: An ovary will ovulate an egg.

The fimbriae will begin to move in such a manner as to draw the ovulated egg into the uterine tube.

Deposit of sperm cells: Sperm cells are deposited at the entrance of the external os of the cervix area.

Sperm enter into the cavity of the uterus.
Sperm enter into the uterine tubes.
Sperm travel about two-thirds of the way down the uterine tube.
If an egg is ovulated and is in the uterine tube, it can be fertilized.
Successful fertilization is at the distal two-thirds of the uterine tube.

Fertilized egg: The fertilized egg is called a **zygote**.

The fertilized egg begins to travel through the uterine tube.
It takes the fertilized egg about seven days to reach the cavity of the uterus.
During this travel time, the endometrial lining becomes thicker to prepare for the implantation of the fertilized egg.
The egg will now implant (bury itself) into the endometrial lining.
A placenta will now form.

UTERINE ATTACHMENT

Look at the figures in your textbook to identify the structures of the female reproductive system that are involved in anchoring the uterus in position.

Anchoring the Uterus

	Structure	Description
1	**Broad Ligament**	This is a huge, flat ligament that covers or surrounds: Anterior and posterior aspects of the uterus. Anterior and posterior aspects of the uterine tubes. Anterior and posterior aspects of the ureters. Anterior and posterior aspects of the ovarian ligaments. This ligament extends from the left pelvic wall to the right pelvic wall and basically sandwiches the uterus in place. The broad ligament splits to cover the anterior uterus and the posterior uterus. This ligament thus forms a partition in the pelvic cavity, forming an anterior cavity and a posterior cavity.
	The broad ligament consists of three main regions:	
2	**Mesometrium**	This is the largest portion that extends from the apical end of the uterus to the inferior edge of the ovary.
	Mesovarium	This is the portion of the broad ligament that covers the ovaries.
	Mesosalpinx	This is the portion of the broad ligament that extends from the superior aspect of the ovary to the uterine tube and covers the uterine tube.

Anchoring the Uterus   (continued)

	Structure	Description
3	Uterosacral ligament	This ligament originates near the entrance to the uterus. It attaches the uterus to the anterior face of the sacrum.
4	Round ligament	This ligament originates inferior to the uterine tube. It eventually connects to the labia majora and mons pubis area.
5	Cardinal ligament	This ligament attaches the lower portion of the uterus to the ischial spines of the pelvis.

Anchoring the Ovaries

	Structure	Description
1	Suspensory ligaments	Also called the **infundibulopelvic ligament** (**IP ligament** or simply **IP**), it connects the ovary to the pelvic wall.
2	Ovarian ligament	This ligament connects the medial portion of the ovary to the uterus near the area of the union of the uterine tubes to the uterus.

FEMALE EXTERNAL GENITALIA

Look at the figures in your textbook to identify the structures of the external genitalia of the female.

Female External Genitalia

	Structure	Description
1	Vulva	This is a term that encompasses all of the external genitalia of the female. The vulva includes: Labia major Labia minora Clitoris Urethral opening (not a part of external genitalia).
2	Vestibule	This is the cavity between the two major folds of the labia minor (labium minus). Within this cavity are: Opening to the vagina Opening to the urethra.
		Beginning at the entrance to the vaginal canal, go lateral (left or right) to identify the following structures: Vaginal canal Leaflets of the **hymen** **Labia minor** (labium minus) **Labia majora** (labium majus)
3	Mons pubis	This is the mound of tissue located at the superior edge of the external genitalia.

1. Fimbriae is Latin that means "fringe."

2. The fimbriae move in such manner as to help draw the egg into the uterine tube.

3. Twins are not due to two sperm cells fertilizing one egg.

    a. The egg consists of 23 chromosomes and the sperm consists of 23 chromosomes. The fertilization of the egg results in a cell with 46 chromosomes.
    b. If 2 sperm cells fertilized the egg, the result would be 69 chromosomes.

4. Fraternal twins are produced when the female ovulates two eggs and each egg is fertilized by a separate sperm cell.

5. Identical twins are produced when the female ovulates one egg and that egg is fertilized by one sperm. Then, the fertilized egg duplicates and splits, thus forming two identical offspring.

6. A tubal ligation is the type of surgery that involves cutting the uterine tubes. Eggs are still ovulated but they cannot traverse the uterine tube.

7. Vagina is Latin that means "sheath."

8. The hymen is a membranous material that partially covers the entrance to the vagina. The rupture or absence of the hymen does not conclusively represent the loss of virginity.

9. Placenta is Latin that means "flat cake."

10. Vulva is Latin that means "covering."

Chapter 9: The Cranial Nerves

This chapter will discuss the cranial nerves. To begin the study of these special peripheral nerves, study the table below.

The Organization of the Nervous System

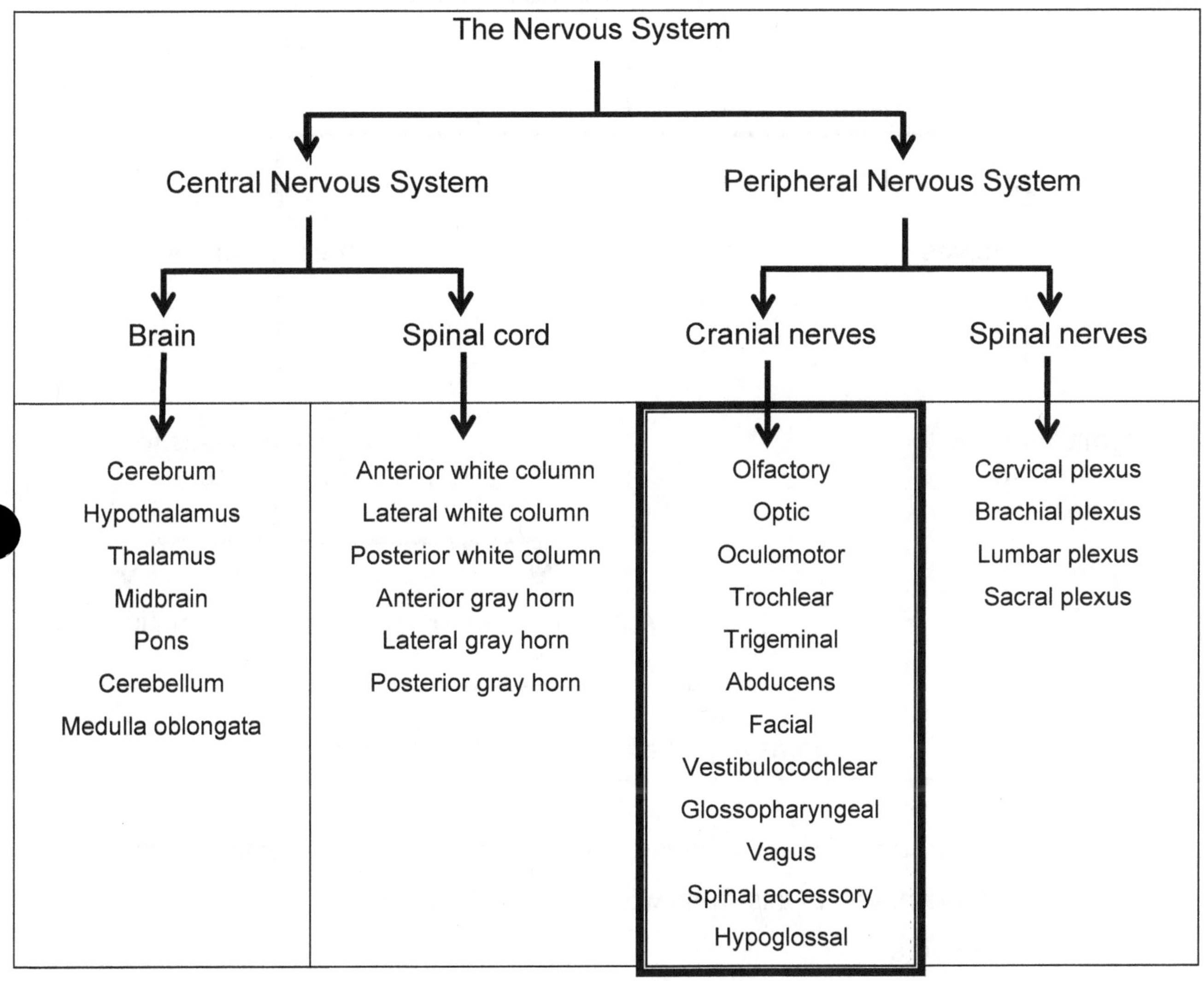

The spinal nerves were discussed in earlier chapters.

The Subdivisions of the Peripheral Nervous System

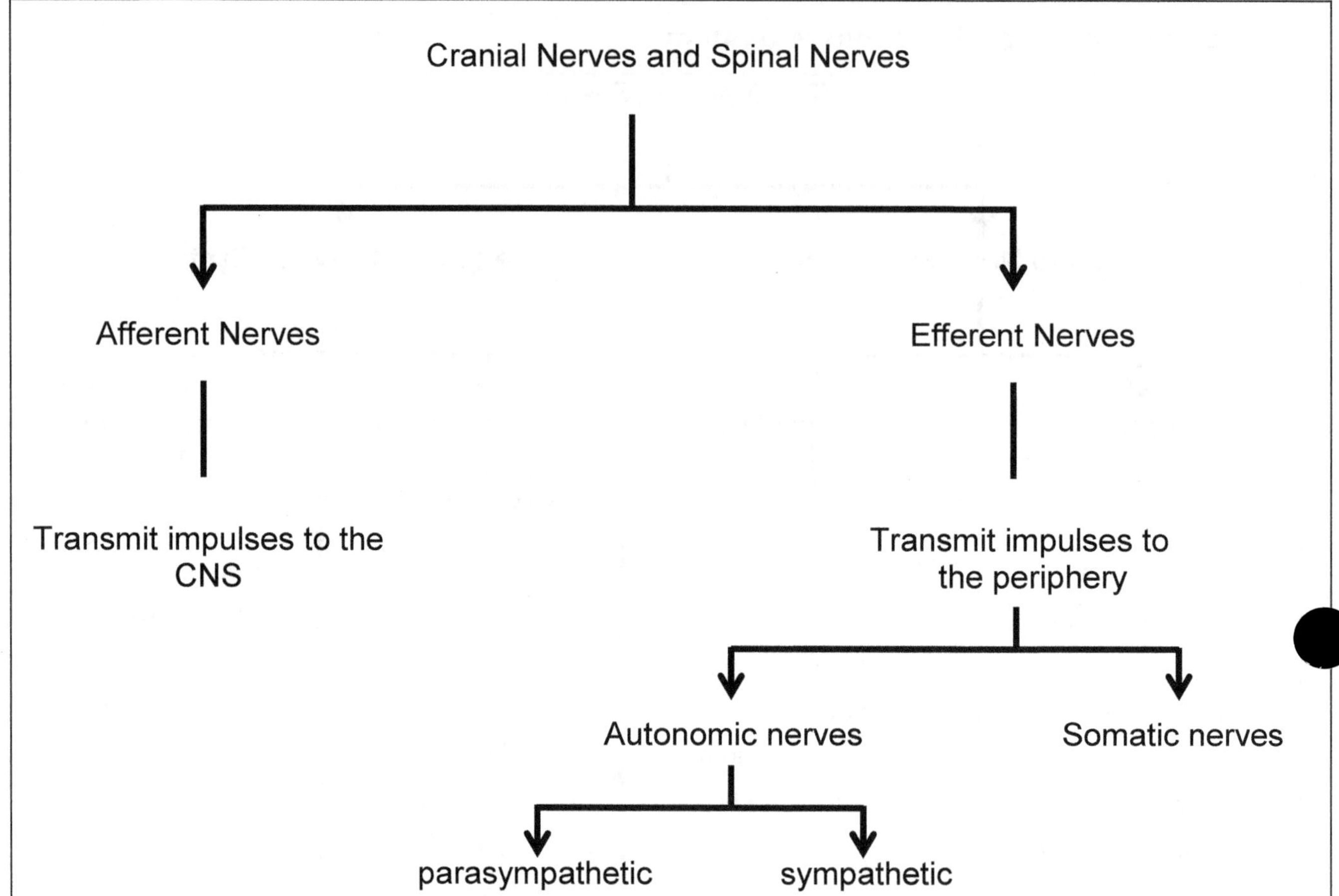

There are 12 pairs of cranial nerves. These nerves are associated with the inferior aspect of the brain. In this class we will study the following:

1. Nerve name
2. Nerve number (Roman numeral)
3. Foramen the nerve passes through
4. Function of the nerve

CRANIAL NERVES

Nerve Number	Nerve Name	Classification	Mnemonic Aid	Nerve Function
I	Olfactory	Sensory	Oh	Senses smell
II	Optic	Sensory	Once	Detects vision
III	Oculomotor	Motor	One	Controls eye muscles for eye movement Controls focusing the lens Pupil constriction
IV	Trochlear	Motor	Takes	Controls superior oblique muscle
V	Trigeminal	Mixed	The	Detects head and face sensations Controls chewing movements
VI	Abducens	Motor	Anatomy	Controls lateral rectus muscle
VII	Facial	Mixed	Final	Detects taste Allows facial expressions
VIII	Vestibulocochlear	Sensory	Very	Senses balance Senses sound
IX	Glossopharyngeal	Mixed	Good	Controls muscles for swallowing Detects tongue sensations
X	Vagus	Mixed	Vacations	Detects thoracic and abdominal organ sensations Controls thoracic and abdominal movements
XI	Spinal accessory	Motor	Seem	Controls trapezius and sternocleidomastoid.
XII	Hypoglossal	Motor	Heavenly	Controls tongue movement

Cranial nerves are also part of the peripheral nervous system. All the nerves of the body are important; but there are 12 pairs of special nerves that are called the 12 cranial nerves. These 12 pairs of nerves are found on the inferior side of the brain. They are organized in sequence beginning at the anterior part of the brain with cranial nerve I (CN I) and ending at the posterior end of the brain with cranial nerve XII (CN XII). The table below introduces some information associated with the cranial nerves.

1	**Motor nerves**	Nerves that transmit impulses from the CNS to the periphery of the body. These are also called **efferent nerves**.
2	**Sensory nerves**	Nerves that transmit impulses from the periphery of the body to the CNS. These are also called **afferent nerves**.
3	**Mixed nerves**	This is a group of nerves that transmits impulses from the CNS to the periphery and also from the periphery to the CNS.

The cranial nerves pass through the various foramina of the skull to arrive at their destinations.

While studying the tables on the following pages, look at the figures in your textbook. Perhaps one way to study the cranial nerves is to study them in separate categories, such as sensory cranial nerves, motor cranial nerves, and mixed cranial nerves.

	Cranial Nerve	Description
I	Olfactory	This nerve transmits sensory information from the nose, through the **olfactory foramina**, to the brain for the interpretation of odor.
II	Optic	The optic nerve transmits sensory information from the eyes, through the **optic canals**, to the occipital lobe of the brain for the interpretation of vision.
VIII	Vestibulocochlear	This nerve transmits information from the cochlea and vestibular apparatus of the ears, through the **internal acoustic canal**, to the brain for the interpretation of sound and balance.

	Cranial Nerve	Description
III	Oculomotor	Transmits motor impulses from the brain, through the **superior orbital fissure**, to control the lens of the eye, the pupil, and it controls all extraocular eye muscles EXCEPT the lateral rectus and the superior oblique.
IV	Trochlear	Transmits motor impulses from the brain, through the **superior orbital fissure**, to control the superior oblique muscle of the eye
VI	Abducens	Transmits motor impulses from the brain, through the **superior orbital fissure**, to control various extraocular eye muscles
XI	Spinal accessory	Transmits motor impulses from the spinal cord, through the **jugular foramen**, to control upper-back and neck muscles
XII	Hypoglossal	Transmits motor impulses from the medulla oblongata, through the **hypoglossal canal**, to control the movement of the tongue

	Cranial Nerve	Description
V	**Trigeminal (ophthalmic portion)**	Transmits sensory information from the forehead, through the **superior orbital fissure**, to the brain for the interpretation of touch
	Trigeminal (maxillary portion)	Transmits sensory information from the maxilla region, through the **foramen rotundum**, to the brain for the interpretation of touch
	Trigeminal (mandibular portion)	Transmits motor impulses from the brain, through the **foramen ovale**, to the masseter muscle for chewing food
VII	**Facial**	Transmits sensory information from the taste buds, through the **internal acoustic canal**, to the brain for the interpretation of taste
		Transmits motor impulses from the brain, through the **internal acoustic canal**, to control the facial muscles and the lacrimal gland of the eyes

	Cranial Nerve	Description
IX	Glossopharyngeal	Transmits sensory information from the tongue, through the **jugular foramen**, to the brain for the interpretation of pain
		Transmits motor impulses from the brain, through the **jugular foramen**, to control the muscles for swallowing
X	Vagus	Transmits sensory information from the thoracic and abdominal organs, through the **jugular foramen**, to the brain for the interpretation of pain. Example: stomach ache.
		Transmits motor impulses from the brain, through the **jugular foramen**, to the thoracic and abdominal organs. Example: slows the heart rate. This is known as a vagal response.

THE CRANIAL NERVES: ADDITIONAL INFORMATION

1. Bell's palsy is an affliction of cranial nerve VII.

2. Many illicit drugs are sympathetic drugs. Many of these drugs cause the pupils to dilate and increase the heart rate.

3. There are three cranial nerves that pass through a foramen, canal, or fissure that has the same name as the opening it passes through.

4. There are two cranial nerves that pass through the internal acoustic canal.

5. There are three cranial nerves that pass through the jugular foramen.

6. There are four cranial nerves that pass through the superior orbital fissure.

7. Damage to the cervical plexus could cause paralysis of the diaphragm muscle.

8. Plexus is Latin that means "to braid."

9. The cranial nerves are numbered (with Roman numerals) from anterior to posterior on the inferior side of the brain.

10. The vagal response is an overstimulation of the vagus nerve (CN X).

Chapter 10: Origin and Insertion of Muscles

Origin and Insertion and Action of Select Muscles

	Muscle name	Origin	Insertion	Action
1	Platysma	Fascia covering the pectoralis major and deltoid	Body of the mandible	Depresses the mandible (opens the jaw)
2	Masseter	Zygomatic arch	Ramus and angle of the mandible	Elevates the mandible (closes the jaw)
3	Rectus abdominis	Pubis area	Ribs 5-7	Flexes vertebral column
4	Erector spinae (iliocostalis)	Iliac crest	Ribs 6-12	Extends vertebral column
5	Biceps brachii (short head)	Coracoid process	Radial tuberosity	Flexion at the elbow
6	Triceps brachii	Proximal end of humerus	Olecranon process	Extension at the elbow
7	Latissimus dorsi	Lower thoracic and all lumbar vertebrae	Intertubercular sulcus of the humerus	Adduction of the arm
8	Deltoid	Acromion process and scapular spine	Deltoid tuberosity	Abduction of the arm
9	Biceps femoris (long head)	Ischial tuberosity	Head of the fibula	Flexion at the knee
10	Rectus femoris	Anterior inferior iliac spine	Tibial tuberosity	Extension at the knee
11	Gastrocnemius	Medial edge of the medial and lateral epicondyles of the femur	Calcaneus	Flexion at the ankle
12	Tibialis anterior	Lateral edge of the proximal portion of the tibia	Metatarsal I	Dorsiflexion at the ankle
13	Gracilis	Inferior portion of pubis	Medial surface of the proximal portion of the tibia	Adduction at the hip
14	Tensor fasciae latae	Lateral edge of iliac crest	Proximal tibia via iliotibial tract	Abduction at the hip

THE FOLLOWING PAGES ARE HOMEWORK PAGES

Chapter 1:   Introductory Terminology

1.   Identify the region between the antebrachium and brachium on the anterior side.

2.   Identify the region between the sural and the femoral region on the posterior side.

3.   Identify the abdominopelvic region that is between the left and right hypochondriac regions.

4.   The cecum of the large intestine can be found in which abdominopelvic region?

5.   What is the term used to describe a condition when a patient has an infection of the left kidney and the spleen?

6. The occipital region is on the _____ side of the head.

7. The hypogastric region is __A__ to the umbilical region. The hypogastric region is __B__ to the inguinal region.

A. ___________________________   B. ___________________________

8. The gluteal fold region is located at the __A__ edge of the gluteus and at the __B__ edge of the femoral area.

A. ___________________________   B. ___________________________

9. The urinary bladder is located in the _____ abdominopelvic region.

10. The philtrum is located __A__ to the nasal septum and __B__ to the center of the upper vermillion border.

A. ___________________________   B. ___________________________

Name _______________________________________

Chapter 2:   Cells and Tissues

1.   What type of muscle do we have control over?

2.   What type of muscle cells are involved in labor contractions?

3.   What type of cells are associated with a matrix called lamellae?

4.   What type of cells provide some degree of protection for the neurons?

5.   Which of the four types of <u>tissue</u> provide us with our first line of defense?

6. Tendons and ligaments are __A__, which means they lack __B__. This allows
the tissue to become more compact, more dense, and therefore real strong. But,
the drawback is due to this, they heal slowly if at all.

A. ______________________________   B. ______________________________

7. Since blood vessels consist of _____muscle, they have the ability to dilate and
constrict automatically.

8. Apply these terms; pseudostratified columnar and simple columnar cells to the
appropriate description.
These columnar cells exhibit nuclei that is arranged at different heights when
comparing one cell to another.

____

These columnar cells exhibit nuclei that are fairly uniform in height when
comparing one cell to another.

____

9. Cardiac muscle and skeletal muscle cells are similar in many ways. However,
the best way to differentiate between cardiac and skeletal muscle is to look for
the presence of _____ in cardiac muscle.

10. Blood technically does not connect anything but it belongs in the connective
tissue category because blood consists of a _____.

Chapter 3:   The Integumentary System

1. Identify the deepest layer of the epidermis.

2. Within which layer of the epidermis can we find the cells that are responsible for creating a tan during the summer time?

3. Which integumentary gland is associated with the formation of acne?

4. What is the name of the integumentary muscles that are involved in creating goose-bumps under certain conditions?

5. When a person is having a manicure and is having their cuticle pushed back, they are actually having what part of the finger nail region pushed back?

6.   How is the integument and sunlight involved in making vitamin D?

7.   Describe what cleavage lines are.

8.   Explain why making a vertical cut in the patella region creates a huge scar but making a horizontal cut in the anterior abdomen creates a small scar that might not even be detectable.

9.   When a child nurses, their nose is pressed up against the areolar region of the nipple and is picking up mom's natural body odor. What integumentary gland is involved in this natural odor from mom?

10. The skin component of the integumentary system helps us to retain heat. However, as we age, we lose heat easily. What is happening to the skin to allow this loss of heat as we age?

Name ____

Chapter 4:   The Skull

1. Identify the superior bony portion of the nasal septum.

2. How many sphenoid and how many ethmoid bones make up the skull?

3. Identify the rounded processes that are on the lateral edge of the foramen magnum.

4. The crista galli is actually the superior tip of what bony process?

5. What is the name of the slanted portion that extends from the dorsum sella to the foramen magnum?

6. Research to determine what specific nerve passes through the foramen rotundum.

7. The __A__ is part of the temporal bone and the __B__ is part of the mandible. These two regions make up the TMJ. The letters, "TMJ" stand for __C__.

A. ____________________________   B. ____________________________

C. ____________________________

8. A. Name the 3 major parts of the sella turcica. B. What major bone of the skull consists of the sella turcica?

B. ____________________________   B. ____________________________

9. The hypoglossal canals form a channel that is on the _____ side of the occipital condyles.

10. Research to find what muscles attach to the styloid processes of the skull.

Chapter 4:   Head and Neck Region --The Muscles

1. The risorius muscle is __A__ to the zygomaticus major and lies on the surface of the __B__ muscle.

   A. _______________________   B. _________________________

2. Place these muscles in the correct sequence going from superior to inferior. Use the letters.

   a.   risorius   b. zygomaticus minor

   c. levator labii superioris alaeque nasi   d. zygomaticus major

   ____________ / ______________ / __________ / ___________

3. Name the three muscles of the chin (that we studied) beginning with the most medial one and going to the most lateral one.

4. Which muscle is more superior to the other:

   zygomaticus minor   or   zygomaticus major?

5. Name the muscles (we studied) that are found between the trapezius and the sternocleidomastoid and list them inferior to superior.

6. Clench your teeth. Put your fingers on the side of your jaw on the muscle that is tensed. Identify that muscle.

7. Some muscles are named, "orbicularis." What does this term mean?

8. Identify five muscles of the head area that have a name that is very similar to the name of the skull bone or bony structure the muscle is located on or attached to.

MUSCLE	BONE OR BONY STRUCTURE

9. What is the name of the material that "connects" the frontalis with the occipitalis muscle?

10. The parotid gland produces an enzyme that begins the process of digestion. What is the name of that enzyme? The parotid duct from that gland lies on the surface of what muscle?

Enzyme: _______________________   Muscle: _______________________

Chapter 4:   Head and Neck Region --The Brain

1. Identify the structure that is located between the thalamus and the pons.

2. Identify the structure that links the two hemispheres of the brain together.

3. Identify the structure that produces cerebrospinal fluid.

4. Identify the specific that produces dopamine.

5. Identify the structure that partitions ventricles one and two of the brain.

6. Put an X over the statement that is NOT correct:

The corpora quadrigemina is posterior to the midbrain.

The corpora quadrigemina is the posterior edge of the midbrain

7. The cingulate gyrus is a major gyrus located _____ to the corpus callosum.

8. Which portion of the cerebral nuclei is located immediately lateral to the lateral ventricles?

9. Which meningeal layer is the most superficial layer of the meninges?

10. The 4th ventricle is between what two prominent brain structures?

Chapter 5:   Upper Appendicular Region --The Bones

1. Which specific part of the clavicle is the conoid tubercle nearest?

2. Identify this condyle: It is a condyle that is located at the distal end of the humerus and slightly medial to the lateral epicondyle.

3. Identify the fossa the head of the humerus articulates with.

4. Identify the bony process that makes up the elbow.

5. Identify the fossa area of the ulna that the head of the radius articulates with.

6. The capitate is located __A__ to the hamate but yet __B__ to the trapezoid.

A. ___________________________   B. ___________________________

7. The dorsal radial tuberosity is located at the __A__ end of the radius on the
    __B__ side.

A. ___________________________   B. ___________________________

8. Identify two parts of the scapula that can be easily palpated.

9. The coronoid fossa is located at the __A__ end of the humerus and is on the
    __B__ side. The olecranon fossa is located at the distal end of the __C__ and is
    on the __D__ side.

A. ___________________________   B. ___________________________

C.___________________________   D. ___________________________

10. Put an X on the statement that is the least correct.

The coronoid process of the ulna is anterior to the trochlear notch.
The coronoid process of the ulna is on the anterior edge of the trochlear notch.

Name _______________________________________

Chapter 5:   Upper Appendicular Region --The Muscles

1. The brachioradialis is the most _____ muscle of the arm.

2. Identify a muscle that is immediately lateral to the palmaris longus.

3. Identify a muscle that is immediately medial to the palmaris longus.

4. Identify a muscle that is between the extensor digitorum and the extensor carpi ulnaris.

5. The tendon of the palmaris longus lies on top of what muscle?

6. Identify all the muscles associated with the rotator cuff.

7. Which part of the biceps brachii is the most medial?

       Long head   or   Short head

8. Which part of the triceps brachii is the most medial?

       Long head   or   Short head   or   Lateral head

9. Which part of the humerus does the flexor digitorum superficialis originate on?

10. The lumbricals and interossei muscles are associated with which aspect of the appendicular skeleton?

Name _______________________________________

Chapter 5: Upper Appendicular Region --The Blood Vessels

1. Blood in the basilic vein will flow into what vein next?

2. Blood in the median cubital vein came from the __A__ vein and will enter the __B__ vein.

    A. ________________________   B. ________________________

3. Blood in the radial and ulnar arteries will flow into what artery next?

4. Blood in the brachial artery will flow into what two arteries next?

    1. ________________________   2. ________________________

5. Blood in the cephalic vein will flow into what two veins next?

    1. ________________________   2. ________________________

6. Which of the following blood vessels is the most medial of the others listed?

Brachial a. / Cephalic a. / Basilic a.

7. Blood in the brachiocephalic artery (trunk) will flow into what two vessels next?

1. ______________________________________

2. ______________________________________

8. Blood in the ulnar artery will flow into what vessel next?

9. Which is deeper; cephalic vein   or   radial vein?

10. What is the name of the artery that "loops" around the humerus near the head of
the humerus?

Chapter 6:   Lower Appendicular Region --The Bones

1. Identify the fossa the head of the femur articulates with.

2. Identify the lateral bone of the lower leg.

3. Identify the large lateral bulge located at the proximal end of the femur.

4. Identify the lateral bulge located at the distal end of the fibula.

5. Identify the tarsal that is lateral to the medial cuneiform.

6. The obturator foramen is located immediately _____ to the acetabulum.

7. The anterior superior iliac spine is the most _____ bulge of the iliac crest. Use a directional term.

8. The intercondylar fossa is __A__ to the lateral condyle and __B__ to the medial condyle. Use directional terms.

A. ____

B. ____

9. The navicular is located immediately _____ to the talus.

10. The medial malleolus is located on the __A__ side of the __B__ (bone).

A. ____

B. ____

Chapter 6:   Lower Appendicular Region --The Muscles

1. Identify the muscles that make up the hamstrings.

2. Identify the muscles that make up the quadriceps.

3. Identify the most medial muscle of the thigh.

4. The biceps femoris muscle is located immediately _____ to the semitendinosus.

5. The tibialis anterior angles a bit to the _____ of the tibia.

medial   or   lateral

6. The adductor magnus is __A__ to the gracilis muscle and the adductor longus is __B__ to the gracilis muscle.

A. ____

B. ____

7. Which of the following is the most lateral muscle of the lower leg?

gastrocnemius   fibularis longus   soleus   tibialis anterior

8. Looking at a lateral view of the leg, put the following muscles in sequence going from posterior to anterior. Use the letters.

a. soleus   b. tibialis anterior
c. fibularis longus   d. gastrocnemius

____________ / ____________ / __________ / ____________

9. The tendons of the fibularis longus and fibularis brevis loop around the:

medial malleolus   or   lateral malleolus

10. The tendons of the tibial posterior and flexor digitorum longus loop around the:

medial malleolus   or   lateral malleolus

Name ____

Chapter 6: Lower Appendicular Region --The Blood Vessels

1. Blood in the femoral artery will flow into what artery next?

2. List the blood vessels in sequence as blood flows from the popliteal vein to the right atrium.

Popliteal v					Right atrium

3. Blood in the great saphenous will enter into what vessel next?

4. Which of the following is true: ___________
   a. The femoral a is anterior to the femur.
   b. The femoral a is posterior to the femur.
   c. The femoral a is medial to the femur.
   d. The femoral a is lateral to the femur.

5. The fibular artery branches off the _____ artery.

6. The medial and lateral plantar artery branches off the ____ artery.

7. The great saphenous is ____ to the femoral vein. Circle your answer.

medial   or   lateral

8. Which of the following arteries pass between the tibia and the fibula? Circle your answer.

Posterior tibial a / Anterior tibial a / Fibular a / Popliteal a

9. Where are the genicular arteries located? Circle your answer.

Tarsal area   Hip area   Middle of the sural area

Knee area   Middle of the femoral area

10. Where are the circumflex arteries located?   Circle your answer.

Tarsal area   Hip area   Middle of the sural area

Knee area   Middle of the femoral area

Chapter 7:   Torso Region --The Bones

1. Identify the muscle that is immediately inferior to the piriformis muscle.

2. Identify the muscle that has a tendon that passes between the two gemellus muscles.

3. Name 7 muscles that insert on the greater trochanter.

1.   3.   5.

                                                                            7.

2.   4.   6.

4. Which of the following is deepest muscle of the ones listed:

        transversus abdominis   /   external oblique   /   internal oblique

5. Which muscle is enclosed by the anterior and posterior rectus sheath?

6. Which muscles of the ribs will cause the ribs to depress during contraction, thereby creating exhalation?

   Internal intercostals   External intercostals

7. The medial portion of the pectoralis major inserts on the ___ (bone structure).

8. Which muscle "lines" the medial aspect of the ilium of the os coxa:

    psoas minor / psoas major / iliacus

9. Which two muscles are combined together to make the iliopsoas muscle?

    psoas minor / psoas major / iliacus

10. There are two major openings in the diaphragm muscle. What structures pass through those two openings?

   Esophagus / Inferior vena cava / Descending aorta

Chapter 7:   Torso Region --The Heart

1. What is the name of the muscular band that extends from the inner lining of the right ventricle to the septum?

2. Identify the opening that exists in the interatrial septum of a fetal heart.

3. Identify the valve that opens into the ascending aorta.

4. Which part of the ECG represents ventricular contraction?

5. Identify the atrioventricular valves of the heart.

6. The pulmonic valve opens into what structure?

7. Oxygenated blood leaves the left ventricle and enters into several arteries, some of which are the coronary arteries. The coronary arteries branch off of the base of what major artery?

8. What structure of the adult heart is being described: This is a structure that holds the aortic to the pulmonary trunk.

9. Which layer of the heart consists of cardiac muscle cells?

10. The coronary sinus is located between the __A__ atrium and the __B__ ventricle on the __C__ side of the heart.

      A. left or right   B. left or right   C. anterior or posterior

Chapter 7:   Torso Region --The Respiratory System

1. Identify the structure that closes over the trachea to prevent choking when swallowing food.

2. What is the anatomical name for the structure known as the "Adam's apple?"

3. Identify the tonsil located in the nasopharynx region.

4. What is the name of the blood vessel that enters the hilum area of the lung?

                Pulmonary artery   or   Pulmonary vein

5. Identify the bronchus that goes fairly straight into the lung as opposed to making a rather "sharp" turn off the trachea.

6. The carina is located at the _____ end of the trachea.

7. The __A__ is cartilaginous tissue that covers the __B__ to prevent choking when a person swallows food.

A. ______________________________   B. ______________________________

8. The palatine tonsils can be seen _____ to the uvula.

9. What is the name of the two cartilaginous pieces located at the proximal end of the trachea?

1. ______________________________   2. ______________________________

10. What is the name of the groove located on the medial-posterior side of the lungs that allows for the entrance and exit of tubes and blood vessels?

Chapter 7:   Torso Region --The Digestive System

1. Identify three salivary glands.

2. Which digestive organ does most of the digestion take place?

3. Enzymes that digest food are produced in the mouth, stomach, small intestine, and _____.

4. The appendix is connected to the _____ of the large intestine.

5. Identify the sphincter that is common between the common bile duct and the pancreatic duct.

6. a. What is the name of the material as it is passing through the esophagus?

    b. What is the name of the material as while it is in the stomach?

      Choices are: bolus or chyme.

    a. ________________________________   b. ________________________________

7. Bile is produced by the __A__ and is stored in the __B__ and will __C__ fat in the __D__.

    A. ________________________________   B. ________________________________

    C.________________________________   D. ________________________________

8. Based on this workbook, how many specific digestive enzymes are **produced** by the following:

    Mouth ________   Stomach ________   Small intestine ________   Pancreas ________

9. Based on this workbook, how many specific digestive enzymes **digest** (or partially digest) material in the following structures:

    Mouth ________   Stomach ________   Small intestine ________

10. The majority of the nutrients are absorbed into the bloodstream via the capillaries that are located in the villi that line the _____.

Name _______________________________________

Chapter 7:   Pelvic Region --The Urinary System

1. Identify the tube that exits the kidneys: _______________________________

    Identify the tubes that exit the urinary bladder: _______________________________

2. Identify the kidney that sits the highest in the body.

3. Identify the tubes that pass through the renal pyramids on their way to the minor
    calyx area.

4. What kind of muscle cells make up the:

    Internal urethral sphincter: _______________________________

    External urethral sphincter: _______________________________

5. Approximately what volume of urine will cause the internal urethral sphincter to
    open?

6. Which urethral sphincter is located at the base of the urinary bladder?

7. Blood in the segmental artery of the kidney enters into what blood vessel next?

8. Blood in the interlobular (cortical radiate) artery will enter into what blood vessel next?

9. Blood in the glomerular capillaries came from what blood vessel?

10. Material in the distal convoluted tubule will enter into what tubule next?

Chapter 8:   Pelvic Region --The Male Reproductive System

1. Identify the tubes inside the testes that are involved in the production of sperm cells.

2. Sperm in the epididymis will swim into what tube next?

3. Identify the muscles that are indirectly involved in helping to maintain proper temperature for sperm development.

4. Identify the reproductive gland that produces the most nutrients for sperm survival.

5. Which tissue of the penis consists of the :

Penile urethra ___________________________________

Arteries ___________________________________

6. List in sequence the muscles that attach the penis to the body beginning with the bulb of the penis and ending with the external anal sphincter muscle.

Bulb of penis				External anal sphincter

7. The crus of the penis are covered by the __A__ muscle, which in turn is attached to the __B__.

A. ___________________________   B. ___________________________

8. Identify the gland that sperm cells enter while swimming through the male reproductive system.

9. Place the following tubes in the order going from the most coiled tube to the least coiled tube: ductus deferens / seminiferous tubules / epididymis

10. The answer to the following questions is either **dartos** or **cremaster**.

A. Which muscle is deeper in reference to the testes? ___________________________

B. Which muscle creates the wrinkles associated with the scrotal sac? ___________

C. Which muscle contracts to pull the testes closer to the abdomen to maintain warm temperatures? ___________________________

Chapter 8: Pelvic Region –The Female Reproductive System

1. Identify the ligament that connects the ovary to the pelvic wall.

2. Identify the ligament that connects the ovary to the uterus.

3. A fertilized egg is called a __A__ and will implant itself in the __B__ of the uterus where it will continue to develop.

   A. ___________________________   B. ___________________________

4. There are numerous hormones associated with the female reproductive system. Research to identify the hormone that is involved in the ovulation of an egg.

5. What kind of muscle cells make up the myometrium of the uterus?

6. Describe where successful fertilization of an egg occurs.

7. The broad ligament is made of three distinct regions. Name them.

1. __________________   2. __________________   3. __________________

8. Place the following in the correct sequence going from anterior to posterior. Put
    a number with each word referencing its sequence.

    ______anus   ______ clitoris   ______vagina   ______ urethral opening

9. Eggs do not have a flagellum like sperm cells have; therefore, what propels the
    egg through the uterine tube?

10. Many books talk about Graafian follicles. What are Graafian follicles?

Chapter 9:   Cranial Nerves

1. Identify which part of CN VIII is involved in hearing and which part is involved in balance.

    Hearing ____________________   Balance ______________________

2. Which portion of the autonomic nervous system causes the pupils of the eyes to constrict when exposed to bright light?

3. Identify (name and number) all of the cranial nerves that are involved in sensory information only.

Number	Cranial nerve name

4. Identify the cranial nerves that have the same name as the foramen or fissure they pass through.

Cranial nerve	Foramen or fissure

5. Identify the cranial nerves that innervate some aspect of the tongue.

6. The affliction of which cranial nerve is involved with Bell's palsy?

7. Name all the cranial nerves involved with controlling the extraocular eye muscles.

1. ___________________   2. ___________________   3. ___________________

8. Describe the "pathway" of the three trigeminal nerves by identifying the following:

Trigeminal nerve branch	origin	foramen	destination
Ophthalmic			
Maxillary			
Mandibular			

9. Which cranial nerve appears to innervate the majority of the thoracic and abdominal organs?

10. Name two cranial nerves that are associated with some aspect of the tongue.